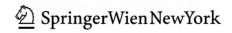 SpringerWienNewYork

W.W. Fleischhacker and D.J. Brooks (eds.)

Neurodevelopmental Disorders

SpringerWienNewYork

Prof. Dr. W. W. Fleischhacker
Department of Biological Psychiatry
Medical University Innsbruck
Anichstrasse 35
6020 Innsbruck, Austria

Prof. Dr. D.J. Brooks
Division of Neurocience and MRC Clinical Sciences Centre
Imperial College, Hammersmith Hospital
Du Cane Road
London W12 0NN, United Kingdom

© 2005 Springer-Verlag/Wien
Printed in Austria

SpringerWienNewYork is a part of Springer Science+Business Media
springeronline.com

Typesetting: Thomson Press India Ltd., New Dehli
Printing: Holzhausen Druck & Medien GmbH, 1140 Wien

Printed on acid-free and chlorine-free bleached paper

SPIN: 11499688

CIP data applied for

With numerous Figures

ISBN-10 3-211-26291-1 (hard cover) SpringerWienNewYork
ISBN-13 978-3-211-26291-7 (hard cover) SpringerWienNewYork
ISBN-10 3-211-26292-X Journal of Neural Transmission [Suppl 69]
(soft cover) SpringerWienNewYork
ISBN-13 978-3-211-26292-4 Journal of Neural Transmission [Suppl 69]
(soft cover) SpringerWienNewYork

Preface

We have great pleasure to present the latest extension of the European Institute of Health Care book series. This volume is devoted to neurodevelopmental disorders. Again, we had the privilege to be able to work with reknowned experts who have agreed to contribute to this endeavour. The book comprises a number of topics related to psychosocial and motor development and is exemplary with regard to its comprehensiveness, as reviews of the topics presented are generally not available in a single publication.

It starts with a timely and critical discussion of the genetics of attention deficit hyperactivity disorder by Dr. Buitelaar in which prospects and challenges of this approach are outlined. The next chapter by Drs. Nicolson and Fawcett deals with dyslexia and its relationship to cerebellar function providing a framework that can explain motor, speed, and phonological deficits in a unified approach. Diagnostic and treatment aspects of speech development disorders are the focus of Dr. Zorowka's contribution in which, among other issues, the necessity of multi-professional cooperation is stressed. Dr. Sigmundsson then focuses on disorders of motor development. 6-10 % of children have motor competence well below the norm, which often persist. The clumsy child syndrome must be seen and treated as a neurological dysfunction. The relationship between tic disorders and obsessive compulsive disorder, two disturbances generally treated by different medical specialists, namely neurologists or psychiatrists, is then reviewed by Drs. Rössner et al. The authors aim to bridge this gap in order to improve diagnosis and treatment. Treatment is also at the core of Dr. Howlin's contribution on children with autism. Following a historical perspective, modern treatment interventions are aptly reviewed and discussed. Lastly, Dr. Remschmidt outlines the problem of childhood and adolescent psychosis covering classification epidemiology and management of these schizophrenia related syndromes.

We hope that you share our enthusiasm for this compilation of expert reviews of an area of medicine that still lacks the widespread interest it deserves.

W. Wolfgang Fleischhacker   **David Brooks**

Contents

Contents

ADHD: strategies to unravel its genetic architecture

J. K. Buitelaar

Department of Psychiatry (333), Radboud University Nijmegen Medical Center,
Nijmegen, The Netherlands

Summary. Attention deficit/hyperactivity disorder (ADHD) is a common and impairing neuropsychiatric disorder with onset at preschool age and strong persistence over time. Its validity as a psychiatric disorder has been established according to Robins and Guze criteria. Genetic factors predominate in the etiology of ADHD. This paper summarizes the current status of genetic research into ADHD, and describes eight factors that complicate research into genetically complex disorders as ADHD. These factors are that multiple genes of small main effects are involved rather than main genes, the relevant phenotype is unknown, presence of clinical heterogeneity, presence of genetic heterogeneity, gene-environment correlation, gene-environment interaction, importance of endophenotypes, and importance of developmental factors. The further unraveling of the genetic architecture of ADHD will depend to a large extent on how well these complicating factors are handled or even used.

Introduction

Attention deficit/hyperactivity disorder (ADHD) is a common and impairing neuropsychiatric disorder with onset at preschool age. It is thought to affect 3–5% of all schoolage children and is characterized by age-inappropriate symptoms of hyperactivity, inattentiveness and impulsivity (American Psychiatric Association, 1994; Buitelaar, 2002). This pattern can be viewed as the extreme of a complex trait that is continuously distributed in the general population and shows a strong overlap with aggressive behavior. The Fourth Edition of the Diagnostic and Statistical Manual (DSM-IV) recognizes three subtypes of ADHD, the predominantly inattentive subtype, the predominantly hyperactive-impulsive subtype and the combined subtype (American Psychiatric Association, 1994). Eighty percent of the children that are diagnosed with ADHD display symptoms in all three domains of inattentiveness, hyperactivity and impulsivity, though at the level of the general population, the inattentive subtype of ADHD is most prevalent (Buitelaar, 2002). There is a much higher incidence rate in boys, who are 1.5–5.8 times more likely than girls to be diagnosed with ADHD (Buitelaar, 2002). The disorder often has a chronic course with about 70% of affected children having threshold ADHD symptoms and associated impairment in adolescence and 30–50% of affected children displaying ADHD symptoms into adulthood (Weiss et al., 1993; Barkley et al., 1990). The presence of comorbid disorders is the rule rather than the exception. Common comorbidities in children and adolescents include oppositional defiant disorder and conduct disorder, anxiety disorders, mood disorders (Biederman et al., 1991), tic disorders, motor coordination disorder (Robinson et al., 1993), learning disabilities (Semrud-Clikeman et al., 1992) and problems in reciprocal social interaction and communication that overlap with those described in autism spectrum disorders (Luteijn et al., 2000a, b). In adolescence and adulthood, comorbid risk taking behaviors and substance abuse disorders are rising in prevalence (Wilens, 2004) as well as antisocial personality disorder (Mannuzza et al., 1989) and borderline personality disorder (Fossati et al., 2002). Numerous problems are further associated over development with ADHD, such as poor academic performance, school drop out, social isolation, and lower occupational success (Weiss et al., 1993; Barkley et al., 1990).

ADHD has been firmly established as a psychiatric disorder that meets the criteria for the validation of psychiatric diagnoses as outlined by Robins and Guze (1970) (Faraone, 2005a). In spite of this, the disorder's validity has been challenged and criticized by popular media, journalists and politicians (Buitelaar and Rothenberger, 2004). ADHD has been stated to be a result of inadequate parenting and teaching in an overstressed society which places to high demands on children's self-control and self-organizational skills. Normal developmental variation and particularly boyish energy and adventurousness have been medicalized. Worries have been further expressed about potential overdiagnosis and overtreatment of ADHD, and particularly on the dangers of the treatment with psychostimulants. Unfortunately, this has led to increase barriers for referral and block access to adequate diagnosis and treatment for children with ADHD and their parents (Buitelaar and Rothenberger, 2004).

The aim of this communication is to summarize the current status of genetic research into ADHD and to describe strategies to further unravel ADHD's genetic architecture.

Behavior-genetic studies

Twin, family, adoption and molecular genetic studies show that genes play a very substantial role in the etiology of ADHD. Family-genetic studies indicate that ADHD aggregates in families, with a 5–8 fold increased risk in first-degree relatives and a 2-fold increased risk in second-degree relatives (Faraone et al., 1994). Twin studies found evidence for a narrow additive heritability of 0.75 to 0.91 which was robust across familial relationships and across definitions of ADHD as the end of a continuum or as a disorder with various symptom cutoffs (Levy et al., 1997; Sherman et al., 1997). For further review of twin studies, see Faraone et al. (2001) and Thapar et al. (1999). Given the modest relative risk ratios in siblings and the fall-off in risk from first to second-degree relatives, the high heritability of ADHD is likely to be due to multiple genes of small effect size (called quantitative trait loci, QTLs, or susceptibility genes) rather than a few genes of major effect. The latter result of the twin studies further indicates that a QTL approach to the study of the genetics of ADHD is valid and that genes associated with a complex trait measure of ADHD very likely will also show to be relevant for ADHD defined as a categorical psychiatric disorder, and vice versa. The fact that heritability is less than 1.0 shows further that features of the environment are also involved in the etiology of the disorder.

Adoption studies of ADHD also implicate genes in its etiology. The adoptive relatives of ADHD children are less likely to have ADHD or associated disorders than are the biological relatives of ADHD children (Morrison et al., 1973; Cantwell, 1975). Biological relatives of ADHD children also do more poorly on standardized measures of attention than do adoptive relatives of ADHD children (Alberts-Corush et al., 1986).

Genome scans

To date, there have been performed three independent genome scans of ADHD. Table 1 summarizes their main results. A first genomewide scan for loci involved in ADHD in 126 affected sib pairs pointed to a number of chromosomal sites that may contain risk factors of moderate effect (Fisher et al., 2002). None of these exceeded genomewide significance thresholds, with LOD scores >1.5 (but <1.66) on 5p12, 10q26, 12q23 and 16p13. The regions containing 29 out of 36 candidate genes, including DRD4 and DAT1, could be excluded for a λ of 2. An extension study in a larger sample of 227 ASPs that focused on chromosome 16q13 was able to establish linkage (LOD score 4.2) (Smalley et al., 2002). A further follow-up investigation extended the original sample of 126

Table 1. Summary of regions implicated in genome scans of ADHD and overlap with regions implicated in other disorders

Study	Region	LOD	Implicated in autism[4]	Implicated in dyslexia[5]
UCLA[1]	5p13	2.6	X	
UCLA[1]	6q12	3.3		
UCLA[1]	16p13	3.7	X	
UCLA[1]	17p11[#]	3.6	X	
Netherlands[2]	15q15	3.5	X	X
Netherlands[2]	7p13	3.0		
Netherlands[2]	9q33	2.1		
Columbia[3]	17p11[#]	2.8	X	
Columbia[3]	11q22	2.5		
Columbia[3]	5q33.3	2.4		

[1]UCLA study of 270 sib-pairs (Fisher et al., 2002; Smalley et al., 2002; Ogdie et al., 2003, 2004)
[2]Dutch study of 164 sib-pairr (Bakker et al., 2003)
[3]Columbian study of 14 three-generation pedigrees (Arcos-Burgos et al., 2004)
[4]For review of genome scans in autism, see Muhle et al. (2004)
[5]For review of genome scans in dyslexia, see Demonet et al. (2004)
[#]Replication of same region

ASPs to 270 ASPs and provided linkage analyses of the entire sample (Ogdie et al., 2003). Maximum LOD score (MLS) analysis identified suggestive linkage for 17p11 and four nominal regions with MLS values 11.0, including 5p13, 6q14, 11q25, MLS p 2.98 and 20q13. These data, taken together with the fine mapping on 16p13, suggested two regions as highly likely to harbor risk genes for ADHD: 16p13 and 17p11. Next, fine mapping was completed of nine positional candidate regions for ADHD in an extended population sample of 308 ASPs (Ogdie et al., 2003). The candidate chromosomal regions were selected from all three published genomewide scans for ADHD, and fine mapping was done to comprehensively validate these positional candidate regions in our sample. Multipoint maximum LOD score (MLS) analysis yielded significant evidence of linkage on 6q12 (MLS 3.30) and 17p11 (MLS 3.63), as well as suggestive evidence on 5p13 (MLS 2.55).

A second genome scan was performed on 164 Dutch affected sib pairs (ASPs) with ADHD (Bakker et al., 2003). Initially, a narrow phenotype was defined, in which all the sib pairs met the full ADHD criteria (117 ASPs). In a broad phenotype, additional sib pairs were included, in which one child had an autistic-spectrum disorder but also met the full ADHD criteria (164 ASPs). This genome scan indicated several regions of interest, two of which showed suggestive evidence for linkage. The most promising chromosome region was located at 15q, with an MLS of 3.54 under the broad phenotype definition. This region was previously implicated in reading disability and autism. In addition, MLSs of 3.04 and 2.05 were found for chromosome regions 7p and 9q in the narrow phenotype. Except for a region on chromosome 5, no overlap was found with regions mentioned in the only other independent genome scan in ADHD reported to date.

The third genome scan was performed in 14 three-generation pedigrees with ADHD from a genetic isolate (Arcos-Burgos et al., 2004). In these families, ADHD is highly comorbid with conduct and oppositional defiant disorders, as well as with alcohol and tobacco dependence. Evidence was found of linkage to markers at chromosomes 4q13.2, 5q33.3, 8q11.23, 11q22, and 17p11 in individual families. Fine mapping applied to these regions resulted in significant linkage in the combined families at chromosomes 4q13, 5q33.3, 11q22 and 17p11. Additionally, suggestive linkage was found at chromosome 8q11.23. Several of these regions were novel (4q13.2, 5q33.3, and 8q11.23), whereas others replicated already-published loci (11q22 and 17p11).

The lack of replication across the studies completed so far adds to the earlier conclusion that genes of moderately large effect are unlikely to exist, and for this reason, further studies are needed to increase the power of available linkage data. Another important outcome of the genome scans is that there appears to be considerable overlap in regions of the genome that are implicated in ADHD, and those that are implicated in other conditions as autism and dyslexia (Table 1).

Candidate gene studies

Numerous candidate genes have been studied for their possible association with ADHD. For more extensive review, see Faraone et al. (2005b). These candidate genes have been chosen to be relevant for current neurobiological theories of ADHD. Many groups have examined associations between

ADHD and genes involved in dopaminergic neurotransmission, mainly because psychostimulants, among the most effective drugs used to treat ADHD, partly block the dopamine transporter (DAT1) function (Volkow et al., 2001; Buitelaar et al., 1995). Dopamine acts also as a agonist at dopaminergic receptor systems. Most studies of the dopamine transporter (DAT1-SLC6A3) gene in ADHD have examined a 10 repeat sequence in the $3'$ untranslated region. When family-based studies of this polymorphism were pooled, the odds ratio is small but significant (1.13, 95% CI 1.03–1.24), suggesting that SLC6A3 merits further investigation but that its effect is modest. One of the best studied candidate genes is the Dopamine D4 receptor (DRD4). Researchers have predominantly focused on a tandem repeat polymorphism in exon III of DRD4 because in vitro studies have shown that one variant (the 7-repeat allele) produces a blunted response to dopamine (Asghari et al., 1995; Van Tol et al., 1992). Despite some variation across studies, when data from analyses of the exon III polymorphism are pooled, the association with ADHD remains statistically significant (case-control odds ratio = 1.45 (95% CI 1.27–1.65); family based OR = 1.16 (95% CI 1.03–1.31). Although the functional implications of mutations in DRD5 are not well understood, there is some evidence for association with long-term potentiation in corticostriatal regions and with locomotion and prepulse inhibition (Manor et al., 2004). A recent analysis that combined 14 independent samples from family-based studies (Lowe et al., 2004) identified a significant association of the 148 bp allele with ADHD, (OR − 1.2; 95% CI 1.1–1.4). Dopamine Beta-Hydroxylase (DBH) is the primary enzyme responsible for conversion of dopamine to norepinephrine. When family-based studies of this gene are pooled, they jointly suggest a significant association between ADHD and the $5'$ Taq1 polymorphism (OR = 1.33, 95% CI 1.11–1.59).

The norepinephrine transporter (SLC6A2) has been examined in ADHD because drugs that block the norepinephrine transporter are efficacious in treating ADHD (Banaschewski et al., 2004). No evidence of association was found for these loci or the haplotypes comprising them in a study that examined SNPs in exon 9, intron 9 and intron 13 in 122 ADHD families and found (Barr et al., 2002). No association with intron 7 and intron 9 SNPs was seen in a study of Irish families (McEvoy et al., 2002), or with a restriction fragment length polymorphism in offspring of adults with ADHD (De Luca et al., 2004).

Serotonin transporter (SLC6A4) is perhaps the best-studied gene in psychiatric genetics, with associations reported for a broad range of diagnoses and traits (Anguelova et al., 2003a, b). When the studies of the 'long' allele of HTTLPR are combined, the pooled odds ratio for the long allele in ADHD samples is 1.31 (95% CI 1.09–1.59). Two family-based association studies examined a silent SNP (G861C) in the gene coding for the serotonin HTR1B receptor. In predominantly Caucasian samples, both studies found over-transmission of the "G" allele, though this finding only reached statistical significance in the very large study which reported pooled results from four sites (Hawi et al., 2002). The association between the over-transmission of the "G" allele and ADHD reached significance as well in a study that analyzed paternal transmission (Quist et al., 2003). The pooled odds ratio for the G861C SNP is 1.44 (95% CI 1.14–1.83).

While these findings on candidate genes are interesting, it is important to note that these genes are of low effect size and explain only approximately 2% of the variance in symptomatology. Further, most of these studies are based on just one of possibly many functional polymorphic variations in specific genes of interest and, unfortunately, most results are inconsistent.

Environmental influences

Before turning to a discussion of the complicating factors in genetic studies, relevant environmental influences will be summarized. Several environmental risks for ADHD have been identified and these are all good candidates for moderation of genetic influences. These environmental risks can be grouped into three categories: 1) pre- and perinatal influences, such as prematurity, low birth weight, pregnancy and birth complications (Hille et al., 2001; Botting et al., 1997; Mick et al., 2002a, b), and mother's use of alcohol or tobacco during pregnancy (Milberger et al., 1996); 2) parental and family factors such as critical expressed emotion versus expressed warmth, inconsistent parenting, parental divorce, family conflict and early institutional rearing (Rutter et al., 2001; Woodward et al., 1998); and 3) acquired neurobiological risks such as closed head trauma and exposure to lead (Thomson et al., 1989; Max et al., 2004; Schachar et al., 2004).

Concerning obstetric adversity, a birth weight lower than 2500 g raises the risk to ADHD about 3–10 times (Breslau et al., 1996; Whitaker et al., 1997). A recent twin study could replicate the association between lower birth weight and increased levels of behavior problems in children as an independent main effect. Interestingly, and in addition, there was an interaction between birth weight and genetic factors in that lower birth weight was associated with decreased genetic influence (Van Os et al., 2001). Obstetric adversity may be co-dependent of the characteristics of the fetus and may mediate genetic risks, as has been shown in the case of autism (Glasson et al., 2004; Bolton et al., 1997). For example, non-affected siblings were more similar to their affected probands than to controls in their profile of birth complications (Glasson et al., 2004). Studies among clinically referred children report particularly high rates of toxemia or eclampsia, maternal illness, maternal psychological stress, bleeding, lengthy labor or delivery, and undue weight loss or gain of the pregnant mother for children with ADHD compared to control children (Milberger et al., 1997; Sprich-Buckminster et al., 1993).

Concerning family functioning, children with ADHD live in a family-environment characterized by marital discord, high rates of parental psychiatric disorder, and low occupation status much more often than controls (Scahill et al., 1999). Family adversity factors as marital discord, low SES, large family size, paternal criminality, maternal mental disorder, and foster placement increased the risk for ADHD and predicted for comorbid disorders, cognitive impairment, and psychosocial dysfunction (Biederman et al., 1995). It is important to appreciate that these associations between family-environment and ADHD are difficult to interpret since a number of these factors such as parental disorder may both reflect genetic transmission and exert an adverse influence through the alteration of parent-child relationships. Further, the family adversities may well be, in part, the consequence of having a problematic child with ADHD rather than the cause of it. Finally, these associations between factors that are defined at the level of the family as a whole, are hard to reconcile with the importance of the nonshared rather than the shared environment, as is shown by twin studies. For example, in an Australian twin study, nonshared environmental influences accounted for about 15% of the variance of ADHD symptoms (Rhee et al., 1999).

Therefore, we will review now work on disrupted parent-child relationships and hyperactivity/aggression. Careful characterization of parent-child relationships of hyperactive children derived from community studies points to the importance of abnormalities of affective tone (especially hostile expressed emotion, HEE) and impairment of parental coping skills (Taylor et al., 1991; Woodward et al., 1998). HHE was seen in 33% of mothers of hyperactive children and in 6% of healthy controls. Poor coping skills were seen in 44% of mothers of hyperactive children and 15% of healthy controls (Woodward et al., 1998). These two sets of figures give odds ratios for the two environmental factors of 7.7 and 3.8 respectively. Hostile parent-child interactions were further found to predict the longitudinal course of children with hyperactivity (Rutter et al., 1997).

Further research is needed to determine whether these are proximal risks effecting the brain directly (e.g. toxicity from alcohol), act indirectly (e.g. maternal drinking correlates with poor parenting and poor parenting is proximal risk), are genetically correlated with the genotype of the mothers (e.g. mothers with ADHD are more prone to smoke during pregnancy than mothers without ADHD) or are genetically correlated with the ADHD proband genotype (e.g. ADHD behavior evokes hostile expressed emotion in the parent).

Complicating factors

Discovering genes involved in ADHD is complicated by several factors (Table 2). The further unraveling of the genetic architecture of ADHD will depend to a large extent on how well these complicating factors are handled and even used. The first one is that the identification of genes of small main effects requires the use of very large sample sizes (Risch et al., 1996). These can only be collected by large consortia, and several of these have been formed over the past years, among which the International Multi-center ADHD GEnetics Project (IMAGE)

Table 2. Complicating factors in genetic studies in complex genetic disorders like ADHD

---

1. Multiple genes of small main effects
2. The relevant phenotype is unknown
3. Clinical heterogeneity
4. Genetic heterogeneity
5. Gene-environment correlation
6. Gene-environment interaction
7. Importance of endophenotypes
8. Importance of developmental factors

Consortium (Asherson, 2004). This consortium under the leadership under Steve Faraone includes more than 10 sites in Europe and aims to collect at least 2000 ADHD families. From these, the 400 most informative concordant pairs and the 400 most informative discordant pairs will be used for initital genomewide linkage studies. Collaborative work has been further facilitated by the ADHD Molecular Genetics Network (NIH grant to Steve Faraone) which comprises investigators from around the world who currently study the genetics of ADHD and meet on a regular basis. A second forum is the EUropean NETwork of HYperactivity DISorders (Eunethydis) (leadership Joe Sergeant) which also has yearly meetings to discuss potential and actual collaboration.

A second factor is that it is unknown on which phenotype molecular-genetic studies should focus. Traditional psychiatric categories as defined in classification schemes as DSM-IV and ICD-10 have been developed for clinical purposes but have not been selected for being relevant phenotypes for genetic research. Twin studies for example indicate that ADHD, and oppositional-defiant/conduct disorder share a substantial amount of genetic factors in childhood (Silberg et al., 1996). There are several approaches to improve the definition of the relevant phenotype for genetic studies. One is based on the work of Risch (1990a, b), who proved that the statistical power of a linkage study increases with the magnitude of risk ratios computed by dividing the affection rate among each relative type (e.g., siblings, offspring) to the rate of affection in the population. These ratio's have been called "lambdas." It was shown that the power depends only on lambda and that defining disease status in a manner that increased lambda would increase the power of linkage studies. According to this logic, Faraone et al. (2000) demonstrated that lambdas were greater if the ADHD proband also has conduct disorder (4.5 and 8.6) and were even greater if the proband has persistent ADHD (17.2 and 19.5). The highest lambdas were found when the proband had both persistent ADHD and CD (25.0–25.9). Another strategy is to fully exploit the potential of twin studies to separate genetic from environmental influences. Though aggregate constructs of ADHD were shown to have heritability as high as 0.80 (see above), similar heritability estimates would not necessarily apply to the single items that are included in these constructs. Twin analyses on single items could afford further information on the decomposition of genetic and environmental influences at the item level, and result in the construction of more "pure" genetically relevant phenotypes. This strategy has been underused sofar. A third strategy is the use of newer multivariate techniques as latent class analysis on ADHD symptoms in twin designs. Such a latent class analysis was applied to data obtained from parents on the 18 DSM-IV ADHD symptoms in 4,036 female twins age 13–23 years in a population sample in Missouri (Todd et al., 2001). The latent-class analysis was most compatible with the existence of three mild and three severe classes of ADHD symptoms in the general population. Unlike DSM-IV subtypes of ADHD, latent-class ADHD subtypes appear to be independently transmitted in families. These classes may be more appropriate targets for molecular genetic studies of ADHD. In another twin dataset the inclusion of sluggish cognitive tempo items markedly changed ADHD symptom associations for boys and girls in a factor analytic framework. In contrast, latent class subtyping of ADHD shows limited impact of the inclusion of sluggish cognitive tempo items, emphasizing the very different assumptions about underlying continua of behavior rather than discrete classes that distinguish the two approaches (Todd et al., 2004). Sofar, latent class subtypes of ADHD have not been used in genetic linkage studies.

Linked to the previous issue of the definition of the phenotype is that of clinical heterogeneity, i.e. that different siblings in a given family may have a different clinical presentation. For example, one sibling may present with one of the ADHD subtypes, whereas another sibling may have dyslexia without ADHD and a third sibling may have autism spectrum disorder (ASD) with comorbid ADHD. The challenges but also opportunities of clinical heterogeneity have not been met addressed sufficiently, particularly in terms of the overlap between ADHD, ASD and dyslexia. Many children with ASD suffer from inattention, hyperactivity and impulsivity to an extent that clinical management of these ADHD-like symptoms is warranted (Handen et al., 2000; Quintana et al., 1995). Re-analyses of the results of population studies on deficits in attention, motor control and perception (DAMP, i.e. a combination of ADHD and perceptual-motor problems) also revealed a strong overlap between severe DAMP and ASD (Kadesjo et al., 1999; Gillberg, 1992). In a similar way, many children with Attention Deficit Hyperactivity Disorder (ADHD) have associated social deficits that are not part of the core symptoms of inattention, hyperactivity and impulsivity that define the disorder. In a study of social disability in ADHD the majority of a sample of 140 boys with ADHD had some degree of difficulty in the social domain (Greene et al., 1996); 22% even qualified as socially disabled, as compared to none of a group of 120 normal controls. In another study, the Children's Social Behavior Questionnaire (CSBQ) was used to compare social deficits in children with ASD, children with ADHD and normal controls (Luteijn et al., 2000a, b). Children with ADHD were characterized by significant social deficits in social interaction and communication and by an increase in stereotypic and restricted behavior, in comparison with normal controls. Although these deficits were significantly more prominent in children with ASD, it appears that there may be an overlap in social deficits between subjects with ASD and ADHD (Luteijn et al., 2000a, b). This all suggests that by subtyping families with (multiple) ASD cases on ADHD characteristics and by subtyping families with (multiple) ADHD cases on ASD characteristics, one can achieve more homogeneous samples and obtain stronger signals in molecular-genetic studies and refine areas of the genome that are implicated in both disorders (Table 1). Similar considerations apply to the subtyping of dyslexia samples for ADHD and of ADHD samples for dyslexia (Loo et al., 2004).

A fourth factor is that of genetic heterogeneity, i.e. different sets of genes may be responsible for risk in different families. This locus heterogeneity may reduce power to detect linkage in traditional affected sibpair studies. On the other hand, the QTLs associated with ADHD are expected to be common genetic variants that are found across human populations (Wright et al., 1999; Risch, 2000). Thus, if population heterogeneity does exist, it is expected to lead to differing prevalence of QTLs in different groups, rather than presence or absence. In ADHD, the prevalence of the DRD4 7-repeat allele, which has been associated with ADHD, varies among populations (Chang et al., 1996). We expect this will be true of other ADHD susceptibility alleles because they are likely to be common alleles, which cause minor, additive deviations in neurodevelopment or neurotransmission. In spite of this, genetic heterogeneity points to the importance of genetic designs which are complementary to affected sibpair designs, such as those using extended 3-generation pedigrees.

Fifth, a full understanding of the genetics of complex behavioral disorders like ADHD will require insights into how environmental risks factors combine with genes to influence the disorder and its clinical features. Some genes might affect ADHD by influencing sensitivity to environmental risks (gene-environment interaction, $G \times E$) or modifying the probability of exposure to environmental risks (gene-environment correlation, rGE). Some other environmental risks may increase susceptibility to ADHD independent of genotype. The potential role of $G \times E$ effects contributing to complex behavioral disorders has recently been demonstrated by two reports from the Dunedin Multidisciplinary Health and Development Study on antisocial behavior and depression in which functional polymorphisms in candidate genes moderated the effects known of environmental stressors, with MAOA moderating the influence of parental maltreatment on antisocial behavior (Caspi et al., 2002) and the serotonin transporter gene moderating the influence of stressful life events on depression (Caspi et al., 2003). Neither of the two genes investigated showed main effects with the behavioral phenotypes in the Dunedin dataset, illustrating the important point that gene associations may be missed if environmental measures are not taken into account. To date, few molecular genetic studies of ADHD have incorporated environmental risk measures. Kahn et al. (2003) found that in pre-school children, hyperactivity-impulsivity and oppositional behavior were associated with the DAT1 10-repeat allele, but only when the child was also exposed to maternal prenatal smoking. Another study explored the possibility of an interaction between the DRD4 gene and season of birth (Seeger et al., 2004). A seasonal pattern of birth has been proposed for different subtypes of ADHD. Therefore, in a subgroup of children with ADHD and conduct disorder, and in healthy controls, children carrying the 7-repeat allele of DRD4 showed different relative risks for developing ADHD and comorbid conduct disorder, depending on the season of birth. This suggests the very likely hypothesis that ADHD, as a multifactorial disorder, may result from variations in genes which have small main effects but whose effects are conditional upon exposure to environmental risk and may be strongly amplified by these environmental risks. If risk exposure differs among participants within a sample, genes may account for little variation in the phenotype. Failure to take account of environmental risk factors in previous genetic studies may be responsible for part of the non-replication results. When exposure to environmental risks differs significantly between samples, candidate genes or regions may fail replication.

An additional strategy is to address heterogeneity at the level of endophenotypes. Endophenotypes are latent traits that are heritable, share genetic loading with the disease phenotype, and are probabilistically related to the disease phenotype as defined in DSM-IV or ICD-10 (Gottesman et al., 2003; Skuse, 2001; Leboyer et al., 1998). These latent traits, which can be measured at a physiological, neurobiological, or cognitive level, may be more closely linked to the underlying genetic factors than the behavioral phenotype and that they

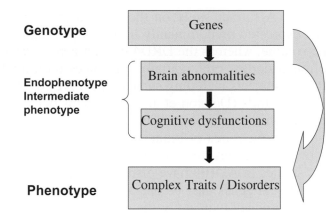

Fig. 1. Outline of the principle of the endophenotype. A smaller set of genes may be involved in the endophenotype than in the complex behavioral trait of clinical disorder

mediate gene-clinical phenotype pathways (see Fig. 1). A smaller set of genes may be involved in the endophenotypes than in the complex behavioral trait or clinical disorder. Endophenotypes may improve the power of molecular genetic studies and may also provide a means of parsing genetic heterogeneity. After many years of searching for one single simple neuropsychological deficit there is a growing realization that ADHD is probably best conceptualized as a neuropsychologically heterogenous condition with differentiable neuropsychological pathways linking specific putative causes to the clinical phenotype (Sonuga-Barke, 2003). These are some studies that suggest that familial ADHD may represent a form of ADHD characterized by a deficient response inhibition. In a study that included ADHD probands with a family history of ADHD, their nonaffected siblings, and normal controls matched for age and IQ, the non-affected siblings were as impaired in measures of response inhibition as the affected probands when compared to the normal controls (Slaats-Willemse et al., 2003). Subjects with ADHD who had a family history of ADHD performed significantly worse on measures of response inhibition than subjects with ADHD without such a family history (Seidman et al., 1995). In addition, children who exhibited poor inhibition (on the stop signal task) were significantly more likely to have a first-degree relative with ADHD than were the children with ADHD who exhibited good behavioral inhibition (Crosbie et al., 2001).

The influence of increased familial risk for ADHD has also been studied on measures of brain morphology (Durston et al., 2004). Both subjects with ADHD and their unaffected siblings displayed reductions in right prefrontal gray matter and left occipital gray and white matter of up to 9.1%. Right cerebellar volume was reduced by 4.9% in subjects with ADHD but not in their unaffected siblings. A 4.0% reduction in intracranial volume was found in subjects with ADHD, while a trend was observed in their unaffected siblings. Thus, the volumetric reductions in cortical gray and white matter in subjects with ADHD were also present in their unaffected siblings, suggesting that they are related to an increased familial risk for the disorder. In contrast, the cerebellum is unaffected in siblings, suggesting that the reduction in volume observed in subjects with ADHD may be more directly related to the pathophysiology of this disorder

(Durston et al., 2004). A further study on the same date-set reported that the DAT1 gene, a gene expressed predominantly in the basal ganglia, preferentially influences caudate volume, whereas the DRD4 gene, a gene expressed predominantly in the prefrontal cortex, preferentially influences prefrontal gray matter volume in a sample of subjects including subjects with ADHD, their unaffected siblings, and healthy controls (Durston et al., 2005). This demonstrates that, by constraining investigations by prior knowledge of gene expression and by using endophenotypes, such as measures of brain morphology, we may begin to map out the pathways by which genes influence behaviour.

Finally, genetic studies in ADHD have disregarded the importance of developmental factors. Different genes may be operating at different ages or developmental stages. In a longitudinal twin study, the relatively high stability of ADHD symptoms over a 5-year period between age 8/9 and age 13/14 year was found. This continuity was mainly due to the same genetic effects operating at both points in time. Change in symptoms between childhood and early adolescence was to a large extent due to new genetic effects in early adolescence but also due to new nonshared environmental effects that became important during adolescence (Larsson et al., 2004). Rather similar results were obtained in another longitudinal twin study which spanned ages 3, 7, 10, and 12 year and used maternal ratings of problem behaviors (Bartels et al., 2004). Stability in externalizing behaviors was accounted for by genetic and shared environmental influences. The genetic contribution to stability for externalizing behaviors was 60% and resulted from the fact that a subset of genes expressed at an earlier age was still active at the next time point. In addition, significant age-specific influences were found for all components, indicating that genetic and environmental factors also contributed to changes in problem behavior. Genetic studies in ADHD should be enriched with a developmental perspective, and explore whether variables as age of onset and severity of disease at various points in time (rather than persistence per se) are relevant developmental endophenotypes.

Concluding remarks

Genetic research of complex disorders like ADHD is one of the most powerful tools to increase our insight into the underlying pathophysiology of the disorder. In the absence of direct neural tissue such as obtained post-mortem or by biopsy, no direct clues as to the neurochemical or cellular or molecular changes at the level of the brain are available. The identification of relevant genes opens new avenues to approach the cellular and molecular base of the disorder. Ultimately, this has the potential to individualize treatment, to facilitate prevention, and to develop new and effective treatments.

References

Alberts-Corush J, Firestone P, Goodman JT (1986) Attention and impulsivity characteristics of the biological and adoptive parents of hyperactive and normal control children. Am J Orthopsychiatry 56(3): 413–423

American Psychiatric Association (APA) (1994) Diagnostic and statistical manual of mental disorders, 4th edn (DSM-IV). APA, Washington DC

Anguelova M, Benkelfat C, Turecki G (2003a) A systematic review of association studies investigating genes coding for serotonin receptors and the serotonin transporter. II. Suicidal behavior. Mol Psychiatry 8(7): 646–653

Anguelova M, Benkelfat C, Turecki G (2003b) A systematic review of association studies investigating genes coding for serotonin receptors and the serotonin transporter. I. Affective disorders. Mol Psychiatry 8(6): 574–591

Arcos-Burgos M, Castellanos FX, Pineda D, Lopera F, Palacio JD, Palacio LG, Rapoport JL, Berg K, Bailey-Wilson JE, Muenke M (2004) Attention-deficit/hyperactivity disorder in a population isolate: linkage to loci at 4q132 5q333 11q22 and 17p11. Am J Hum Genet 75(6): 998–1014

Asghari V, Sanyal S, Buchwaldt S, Paterson A, Jovanovic V, Van Tol HH (1995) Modulation of intracellular cyclic AMP levels by different human dopamine D4 receptor variants. J Neurochem 65(3): 1157–1165

Asherson P (2004) Attention-Deficit Hyperactivity Disorder in the post-genomic era. Eur Child Adolesc Psychiatry 13 [Suppl 1]: I50–I70

Bakker SC, van der Meulen EM, Buitelaar JK, Sandkuijl LA, Pauls DL, Monsuur AJ, Slot RvR, Minderaa RB, Gunning WB, Pearson PL, Sinke RJ (2003) A whole-genome scan in 164 dutch sib pairs with attention-deficit/hyperactivity disorder: suggestive evidence for linkage on chromosomes 7p and 15q. Am J Hum Genet 72(5): 1251–1260

Banaschewski T, Roessner V, Dittmann RW, Santosh PJ, Rothenberger A (2004) Non-stimulant medications in the treatment of ADHD. Eur Child Adolesc Psychiatry 13 [Suppl 1]: 102–116

Barkley RA, Fischer M, Edelbrock CS, Smallish L (1990) The adolescent outcome of hyperactive children diagnosed by research criteria. I. An 8-year prospective follow-up study. J Am Acad Child Adolesc Psychiatry 29(4): 546–557

Barr CL, Kroft J, Feng Y, Wigg K, Roberts W, Malone M, Ickowicz A, Schachar R, Tannock R, Kennedy JL (2002) The norepinephrine transporter gene and attention-deficit hyperactivity disorder. Am J Med Genet 114(3): 255–259

Bartels M, Van Den Oord EJ, Hudziak JJ, Rietveld MJ, van Beijsterveldt CE, Boomsma DI (2004) Genetic and environmental mechanisms underlying stability and change in problem behaviors at ages 3 7 10 and 12. Dev Psychol 40(5): 852–867

Biederman J, Newcorn J, Sprich S (1991) Comorbidity of attention deficit hyperactivity disorder with conduct depressive anxiety and other disorders. Am J Psychiatry 148: 564–577

Biederman J, Milberger S, Faraone SV, Kiely K, Guite J, Mick E, Ablon S, Warburton R, Reed E (1995) Family-environment risk factors for attention-deficit hyperactivity disorder. A test of Rutter's indicators of adversity. Arch Gen Psychiatry 52: 464–470

Bolton PF, Murphy M, Macdonald H, Whitlock B, Pickles A, Rutter M (1997) Obstetric complications in autism: consequences or causes of the condition? J Am Acad Child Adolesc Psychiatry 36(2): 272–281

Botting N, Powls A, Cooke RWI (1997) Attention Deficit Hyperactivity Disorders and other psychiatric outcomes in very low birth weight children at 12 years. J Child Psychol Psychiatry 38: 931–941

Breslau N, Brown GG, DelDotto JE, Kumar S, Ezhuthachan S, Andreski P, Hufnagle KG (1996) Psychiatric sequelae of low birth weight at 6 years of age. J Abnorm Child Psychol 24(3): 385–400

Buitelaar JK (2002) Epidemiological aspects: what have we learned over the last decade? In: Sandberg S (ed) Hyperactivity and attention disorders of childhood, 2nd edn. Cambridge University Press, Cambridge, pp 30–63

Buitelaar JK, Rothenberger A (2004) Foreword – ADHD in the scientific and political context. Eur Child Adolesc Psychiatry 13 [Suppl 1]: 1–6

Buitelaar JK, Van der Gaag RJ, Swaab-Barneveld H, Kuiper M, Van Engeland H (1995) Prediction of clinical response to methylphenidate in children with attention-deficit hyperactivity disorder (abstract). Proc 10th ESCAP Congress 10: 92–93

Cantwell DP (1975) Genetics of hyperactivity. J Child Psychol Psychiatr Allied Disciplines 16(3): 261–264

Caspi A, McClay J, Moffitt TE, Mill J, Martin J, Craig IW, Taylor A, Poulton R (2002) Role of genotype in the cycle of violence in maltreated children. Science 297: 851–854

Caspi A, Sugden K, Moffitt TE, Taylor A, Craig IW, Harrington H, McClay J, Mill J, Martin J, Braithwaite A, Poulton R (2003) Influence of life stress on depression: moderation by a polymorphism in the 5-HTT gene. Science 301(5631): 386–389

Chang FM, Kidd JR, Livak KJ, Pakstis AJ, Kidd KK (1996) The world-wide distribution of allele frequencies at the human dopamine D4 receptor locus. Hum Genet 98(1): 91–101

Crosbie J, Schachar R (2001) Deficient inhibition as a marker for familial ADHD. Am J Psychiatry 158(11): 1884–1890

De Luca V, Muglia P, Vincent JB, Lanktree M, Jain U, Kennedy JL (2004) Adrenergic alpha 2C receptor genomic organization: association study in adult ADHD. Am J Med Genet B Neuropsychiatr Genet 127(1): 65–67

Demonet JF, Taylor MJ, Chaix Y (2004) Developmental dyslexia. Lancet 363(9419): 1451–1460

Durston S, Hulshoff Pol HE, Schnack HG, Buitelaar JK, Steenhuis MP, Minderaa RB, Kahn RS, Van Engeland H (2004) Magnetic resonance imaging of boys with attention-deficit/hyper-hyperactivity disorder and their unaffected siblings. J Am Acad Child Adolesc Psychiatry 43(3): 332–340

Durston S, Fossella JA, Casey BJ, Hulshoff Pol HE, Galvan A, Schnack HG, Steenhuis MP, Minderaa RB, Buitelaar JK, Kahn RS, Van Engeland H (2005) Differential effects of DRD4 and DAT1 genotype on fronto-striatal gray matter volumes in a sample of subjects with attention deficit hyperactivity disorder their unaffected siblings and controls. Mol Psychiatry 10(7): 678–685

Faraone SV (2005a) The scientific foundation for understanding attention-deficit/hyperactivity disorder as a valid psychiatric disorder. Eur Child Adolesc Psychiatr 14(1): 1–10

Faraone SV, Perlis RH, Doyle AE, Smoller JW, Goralnick JJ, Holmgren MA, Sklar P (2005b) Molecular genetics of attention deficit hyperactivity disorder. Biol Psychiatry 57(11): 1313–1323

Faraone SV, Biederman J (1994) Genetics of attention-deficit hyperactivity disorder. Child Adolesc Psychiatr Clin N Am 3: 285–302

Faraone SV, Doyle AE (2001) The nature and heritability of attention-deficit/hyperactivity disorder. Child Adolesc Psychiatr Clin N Am 10(2): 299–316 viii–ix

Faraone SV, Biederman J, Monuteaux MC (2000) Toward guidelines for pedigree selection in genetic studies of Attention Deficit Hyperactivity Disorder. Genet Epidemiol 18: 1–16

Fisher SE, Francks C, McCracken JT, McGough JJ, Marlow AJ, Macphie IL, Newbury DF, Crawford LR, Palmer CG, Woodward JA, Del'Homme M, Cantwell DP, Nelson SF, Monaco AP, Smalley SL (2002) A genomewide scan for loci involved in attention-deficit/hyperactivity disorder. Am J Hum Genet 70(5): 1183–1196

Fossati A, Novella L, Donati D, Donini M, Maffei C (2002) History of childhood attention deficit/hyperactivity disorder symptoms and borderline personality disorder: a controlled study. Compr Psychiatry 43(5): 369–377

Gillberg CL (1992) Autism and autistic-like conditions – subclasses among disorders of empathy. J Child Psychol Psychiat 33: 813–842

Glasson EJ, Bower C, Petterson B, de Klerk N, Chaney G, Hallmayer JF (2004) Perinatal factors and the development of autism: a population study. Arch Gen Psychiatry 61(6): 618–627

Gottesman II, Gould TD (2003) The endophenotype concept in psychiatry: etymology and strategic intentions. Am J Psychiatry 160(4): 636–645

Greene RW, Biederman J, Faraone SV, Ouellette CA, Penn C, Griffin SM (1996) Toward a new psychometric definition of social disability in children with attention-deficit hyperactivity disorder. J Am Acad Child Adolesc Psychiatry 35(5): 571–578

Handen BL, Johnson CR, Lubetsky MJ (2000) Efficacy of methylphenidate among children with autism and symptoms of attention-deficit hyperactivity disorder. J Autism Dev Disord 30: 245–255

Hawi Z, Dring M, Kirley A, Foley D, Kent L, Craddock N, Asherson P, Curran S, Gould A, Richards S, Lawson D, Pay H, Turic D, Langley K, Owen M, O'Donovan M, Thapar A, Fitzgerald M, Gill M (2002) Serotonergic system and attention deficit hyperactivity disorder (ADHD): a potential susceptibility locus at the 5-HT(1B) receptor gene in 273 nuclear families from a multi-centre sample. Mol Psychiatry 7(7): 718–725

Hille ET, den Ouden AL, Saigal S, Wolke D, Lambert M, Whitaker A, Pinto-Martin JA, Hoult L, Meyer R, Feldman JF, Verloove-Vanhorick SP, Paneth N (2001) Behavioural problems in children who weigh 1000 g or less at birth in four countries. Lancet 357(9269): 1641–1643

Kadesjo B, Gillberg C, Hagberg B (1999) Brief report: autism and Asperger syndrome in seven-year-old children: a total population study. J Autism Dev Disord 29(4): 327–331

Kahn RS, Khoury J, Nichols WC, Lanphear BP (2003) Role of dopamine transporter genotype and maternal prenatal smoking in childhood hyperactive-impulsive inattentive and oppositional behaviors. J Pediatr 143(1): 104–110

Larsson JO, Larsson H, Lichtenstein P (2004) Genetic and environmental contributions to stability and change of ADHD symptoms between 8 and 13 years of age: a longitudinal twin study. J Am Acad Child Adolesc Psychiatry 43(10): 1267–1275

Leboyer M, Bellivier F, Nosten-Bertrand M, Jouvent R, Pauls D, Mallet J (1998) Psychiatric genetics: search for phenotypes. Trends Neurosci 21(3): 102–105

Levy F, Hay DA, McStephen M, Wood C, Waldman I (1997) Attention-deficit hyperactivity disorder: a category or a continuum? Genetic analysis of a large-scale twin study. J Am Acad Child Adolesc Psychiatry 36(6): 737–744

Loo SK, Fisher SE, Francks C, Ogdie MN, Macphie IL, Yang M, McCracken JT, McGough JJ, Nelson SF, Monaco AP, Smalley SL (2004) Genome-wide scan of reading ability in affected sibling pairs with attention-deficit/hyperactivity disorder: unique and shared genetic effects. Mol Psychiatry 9(5): 485–493

Lowe N, Kirley A, Hawi Z, Sham P, Wickham H, Kratochvil CJ, Smith SD, Lee SY, Levy F, Kent L, Middle F, Rohde LA, Roman T, Tahir E, Yazgan Y, Asherson P, Mill J, Thapar A, Payton A, Todd RD, Stephens T, Ebstein RP, Manor I, Barr CL, Wigg KG, Sinke RJ, Buitelaar JK, Smalley SL, Nelson SF, Biederman J, Faraone SV, Gill M (2004) Joint analysis of the DRD5 marker concludes association with Attention-Deficit/Hyperactivity Disorder confined to the predominantly inattentive and combined subtypes. Am J Hum Genet 74(2): 348–356

Luteijn E, Luteijn F, Jackson S, Volkmar F, Minderaa R (2000a) The children's Social Behavior Questionnaire for milder variants of PDD problems: evaluation of the psychometric characteristics. J Autism Dev Disord 30(4): 317–330

Luteijn EF, Serra M, Jackson S, Steenhuis MP, Althaus M, Volkmar F, Minderaa R (2000b) How unspecified are disorders of children with a pervasive developmental disorder not otherwise specified? A study of social problems in children with PDD-NOS and ADHD. Eur Child Adolesc Psychiatry 9(3): 168–179

Mannuzza S, Gittelman Klein R, Horowitz Konig P, Giampino TL (1989) Hyperactive boys almost grown up. IV. Criminality and its relationship to psychiatric status. Arch Gen Psychiatry 46: 1073–1079

Manor I, Corbex M, Eisenberg J, Gritsenkso I, Bachner-Melman R, Tyano S, Ebstein RP (2004) Association of the dopamine D5 receptor with attention deficit hyperactivity disorder (ADHD) and scores on a continuous performance test (TOVA). Am J Med Genet B Neuropsychiatr Genet 127(1): 73–77

Max JE, Lansing AE, Koele SL, Castillo CS, Bokura H, Schachar R, Collings N, Williams KE (2004) Attention deficit hyperactivity disorder in children and adolescents following traumatic brain injury. Dev Neuropsychol 25(1–2): 159–177

McEvoy B, Hawi Z, Fitzgerald M, Gill M (2002) No evidence of linkage or association between the norepinephrine transporter (NET) gene polymorphisms and ADHD in the Irish population. Am J Med Genet 114(6): 665–666

Mick E, Biederman J, Faraone SV, Sayer J, Kleinman S (2002a) Case-control study of attention-deficit hyperactivity disorder and maternal smoking alcohol use and drug use during pregnancy. J Am Acad Child Adolesc Psychiatry 41(4): 378–385

Mick E, Biederman J, Prince J, Fischer MJ, Faraone SV (2002b) Impact of low birth weight on attention-deficit hyperactivity disorder. J Dev Behav Pediatr 23(1): 16–22

Milberger S, Biederman J, Faraone SV, Chen L, Jones J (1996) Is maternal smoking during pregnancy a risk factor for attention deficit hyperactivity disorder in children? [see comments] Am J Psychiatry 153(9): 1138–1142

Milberger S, Biederman J, Faraone SV, Guite J, Tsuang MT (1997) Pregnancy delivery and infancy complications and attention deficit hyperactivity disorder: issues of gene-environment interaction. Biol Psychiatry 41(1): 65–75

Morrison JR, Stewart MA (1973) The psychiatric status of the legal families of adopted hyperactive children. Arch Gen Psychiatry 28(6): 888–891

Muhle R, Trentacoste SV, Rapin I (2004) The genetics of autism. Pediatrics 113(5): e472–486

Ogdie MN, Macphie IL, Minassian SL, Yang M, Fisher SE, Francks C, Cantor RM, McCracken JT, McGough JJ, Nelson SF, Monaco AP, Smalley SL (2003) A genomewide scan for attention-deficit/hyperactivity disorder in an extended sample: suggestive linkage on 17p11. Am J Hum Genet 72(5): 1268–1279

Quintana H, Birmaher B, Stedge D, Lennon S, Freed J, Bridge J, Greenhill L (1995) Use of methylphenidate in the treatment of children with autistic disorder. J Autism Dev Disord 25(3): 283–294

Quist JF, Barr CL, Schachar R, Roberts W, Malone M, Tannock R, Basile VS, Beitchman J, Kennedy JL (2003) The serotonin 5-HT1B receptor gene and attention deficit hyperactivity disorder. Mol Psychiatry 8(1): 98–102

Rhee SH, Waldman ID, Hay DA, Levy F (1999) Sex differences in genetic and environmental influences on DSM-III-R attention-deficit/hyperactivity disorder. J Abnorm Psychol 108(1): 24–41

Risch N (1990a) Linkage strategies for genetically complex traits. II. The power of affected relative pairs. Am J Hum Genet 46(2): 229–241

Risch N (1990b) Linkage strategies for genetically complex traits. I. Multilocus models. Am J Hum Genet 46(2): 222–228

Risch NJ (2000) Searching for genetic determinants in the new millennium. Nature 405(6788): 847–856

Risch NJ, Zhang H (1996) Mapping quantitative trait loci with extreme discordant sib pairs: sampling considerations. Am J Hum Genet 58(4): 836–843

Robins E, Guze SB (1970) Establishment of diagnostic validity in psychiatric illness: its application to schizophrenia. Am J Psychiatry 126(7): 983–987

Robinson WP, Wagstaff J, Bernasconi F, Baccichetti C, Artifoni L, Franzoni E, Suslak L, Shih LY, Aviv H, Schinzel AA (1993) Uniparental disomy explains the occurrence of the Angelman or Prader-Willi syndrome in patients with an additional small inv dup(15) chromosome. J Med Genet 30(9): 756–760

Rutter M, Maughan B, Meyer J, Pickles A, Silberg J, Simonoff E, Taylor E (1997) Heterogeneity of antisocial behavior: causes continuities and consequences. Nebr Symp Motiv 44: 45–118

Rutter ML, Kreppner JM, O'Connor TG (2001) Specificity and heterogeneity in children's responses to profound institutional privation. Br J Psychiatry 179: 97–103

Scahill L, Schwab-Stone ME, Merikangas KR, Leckman JF, Zhang H, Kasl S (1999) Psycho-social and clinical correlates of ADHD in a community sample of school-age children. J Am Acad Child Adolesc Psychiatry 38(8): 976–984

Schachar R, Levin HS, Max JE, Purvis K, Chen S (2004) Attention deficit hyperactivity disorder symptoms and response inhibition after closed head injury in children: do preinjury behavior and injury severity predict outcome? Dev Neuropsychol 25(1–2): 179–198

Seeger G, Schloss P, Schmidt MH, Ruter-Jungfleisch A, Henn FA (2004) Gene-environment interaction in hyperkinetic conduct disorder (HD + CD) as indicated by season of birth variations in dopamine receptor (DRD4) gene polymorphism. Neurosci Lett 366(3): 282–286

Seidman LJ, Biederman J, Faraone SV, Milberger S, Norman D, Seiverd K, Benedict K, Guite J, Mick E, Kiely K (1995) Effects of family history and comorbidity on the neuropsychological performance of children with ADHD: preliminary findings. J Am Acad Child Adolesc Psychiatry 34(8): 1015–1024

Semrud-Clikeman M, Biederman J, Sprich-Buckminster S, Lehman BK, Faraone SV, Norman D (1992) Comorbidity between ADDH and learning disability: a review and report in a clinically referred sample. J Am Acad Child Adolesc Psychiatry 31(3): 439–448

Sherman DK, Iacono WG, McGue MK (1997) Attention-deficit hyperactivity disorder dimensions: a twin study of inattention and impulsivity-hyperactivity. J Am Acad Child Adolesc Psychiatry 36(6): 745–753

Silberg J, Rutter M, Meyer J, Maes H, Hewitt J, Simonoff E, Pickles A, Loeber R, Eaves L (1996) Genetic and environmental influences on the covariation between hyperactivity and conduct disturbance in juvenile twins. J Child Psychol Psychiatry 37(7): 803–816

Skuse DH (2001) Endophenotypes and child psychiatry. Br J Psychiatry 178: 395–396

Slaats-Willemse DIE, Swaab-Barneveld H, De Sonneville LMJ, van der Meulen EM, Buitelaar JK (2003) Deficient response inhibition as a cognitive endophenotype of ADHD. J Am Acad Child Adolesc Psychiatry 42: 1242–1248

Smalley SL, Kustanovich V, Minassian SL, Stone JL, Ogdie MN, McGough JJ, McCracken JT, Macphie IL, Francks C, Fisher SE, Cantor RM, Monaco AP, Nelson SF (2002) Genetic linkage of attention-deficit/hyperactivity disorder on chromosome 16p13 in a region implicated in autism. Am J Hum Genet 71(4): 959–963

Sonuga-Barke EJ (2003) The dual pathway model of AD/HD: an elaboration of neuro-developmental characteristics. Neurosci Biobehav Rev 27(7): 593–604

Sprich-Buckminster S, Biederman J, Milberger S, Faraone SV, Lehman BK (1993) Are perinatal complications relevant to the manifestation of ADD? Issues of comorbidity and familiality. J Am Acad Child Adolesc Psychiatry 32(5): 1032–1037

Taylor E, Sandberg S, Thorley G, Giles S (1991) The epidemiology of hyperactivity. Oxford University Press, Oxford

Thapar A, Holmes J, Poulton K, Harrington R (1999) Genetic basis of attention deficit and hyperactivity. Br J Psychiatry 174: 105–111

Thomson GOB, Raab GM, Hepburn WS, Hunter R, Fulton M, Laxen DPH (1989) Lood-lead levels and children's behavior: results from the Edinburgh lead study. J Child Psychol Psychiat 30: 515–528

Todd RD, Rasmussen ER, Neuman RJ, Reich W, Hudziak JJ, Bucholz KK, Madden PA, Heath A (2001) Familiality and heritability of subtypes of attention deficit hyperactivity disorder in a population sample of adolescent female twins. Am J Psychiatry 158(11): 1891–1898

Todd RD, Rasmussen ER, Wood C, Levy F, Hay DA (2004) Should sluggish cognitive tempo symptoms be included in the diagnosis of attention-deficit/hyperactivity disorder? J Am Acad Child Adolesc Psychiatry 43(5): 588–597

Van Os J, Wichers M, Danckaerts M, Van Gestel S, Derom C, Vlietinck R (2001) A prospective twin study of birth weight discordance and child problem behavior. Biol Psychiatry 50(8): 593–599

Van Tol HH, Wu CM, Guan HC, Ohara K, Bunzow JR, Civelli O, Kennedy J, Seeman P, Niznik HB, Jovanovic V (1992) Multiple dopamine D4 receptor variants in the human population. Nature 358: 149–152

Volkow ND, Wang G, Fowler JS, Logan J, Gerasimov M, Maynard L, Ding Y, Gatley SJ, Gifford A, Franceschi D (2001) Therapeutic doses of oral methylphenidate significantly increase extracellular dopamine in the human brain. J Neurosci 21(2): RC121

Weiss G, Hechtman L (1993) Hyperactive childen grown up ADHD in children adolescents and adults, 2nd ed. Guilford Press, New York

Whitaker AH, Van Rossum R, Feldman JF, Schonfeld IS, Pinto-Martin JA, Torre C, Shaffer D, Paneth N (1997) Psychiatric outcomes in low-birth-weight children at age 6 years: relation to neonatal cranial ultrassound abnormalities. Arch Gen Psychiatry 54: 847–856

Wilens TE (2004) Attention-deficit/hyperactivity disorder and the substance use disorders: the nature of the relationship subtypes at risk and treatment issues. Psychiatr Clin N Am 27(2): 283–301

Woodward L, Taylor E, Dowdney L (1998) The parenting and family functioning of children with hyperactivity. J Child Psychol Psychiatr Allied Disciplines 39(2): 161–169

Wright AF, Carothers AD, Pirastu M (1999) Population choice in mapping genes for complex diseases. Nat Genet 23(4): 397–404

Author's address: J. K. Buitelaar, Department of Psychiatry (333), Radboud University Nijmegen Medical Center, P.O. Box 9101, 6500 HB Nijmegen, The Netherlands, e-mail: J.Buitelaar@psy.umcn.nl

Developmental dyslexia, learning and the cerebellum

R. I. Nicolson and **A. J. Fawcett**

Department of Psychology, University of Sheffield, Sheffield, United Kingdom

Summary. Theoretical frameworks for dyslexia must explain how the well-established phonological deficits and the literacy deficits arise. Our longstanding research programme has led to a distinctive 'twin level' framework that proposes, first, that the core deficits are well described in terms of poor skill automaticity. Second, these 'cognitive level' symptoms are attributed to abnormal cerebellar function – a 'brain-level' analysis. The evidence includes data from behavioural, imaging, neuroanatomical and learning studies. The framework leads to an 'ontogenetic' analysis that links cerebellar deficit at birth, via problems in articulation and working memory, to the known phonological, speed and literacy difficulties. Differences in locus of cerebellar impairment, experience and/or links to other brain regions may account for subtypes of dyslexia and possibly other developmental disorders. The automaticity/cerebellar deficit framework provides an explicit demonstration that it is possible to explain motor, speed and phonological deficits within a unified account, integrating previously opposed approaches.

Specific developmental dyslexia is normally characterised by unexpected problems in learning to read for children of average or above average intelligence. It is arguably the major developmental disorder, with a prevalence in Western societies of at least 4% (Badian, 1984; Jorm et al., 1986). One of the major challenges for dyslexia research is to establish frameworks sufficiently general and sufficiently integrated to account for dyslexia from theoretical, diagnostic and remedial perspectives. From a theoretical perspective a framework should ideally be grounded at biological, cognitive and behavioural levels of description. From a remedial perspective, a framework should be able to adapt to individual symptoms, and provide support both for age-appropriate literacy and life skills. Diagnosis should provide the bridge between theory and remediation, providing the means by which theoretically-derived diagnostic data inform the design of that individual's remediation programmes. In this paper we present an integrated theoretical analysis that might provide a useful starting place for the development of such a unified framework. First, however, it is valuable to give some background information.

There is still considerable debate over diagnostic methods, but a standard criterion is *"a disorder in children who, despite conventional classroom experience, fail to attain the language skills of reading, writing and spelling commensurate with their intellectual abilities"* (World Federation of Neurology, 1968). It has been assumed that the problems of dyslexic children derive from impairment of some skill or cognitive component largely specific to the reading process, and one of the major achievements of dyslexia research in the past decades was the demonstration that many of the reading-related deficits may be attributed to some disorder of phonological processing (Vellutino, 1979; Bradley and Bryant, 1983; Snowling, 1987; Stanovich, 1988; Shankweiler et al., 1995).

Although there is no doubt that difficulties in processing phonological information are a characteristic feature of dyslexia, phonological difficulties can arise from a wide range of causes, and arguably the key theoretical priority for dyslexia research is to identify the underlying cause(s) of the phonological deficits. For these purposes it is important to establish the full range of symptoms of dyslexia (whether or not they are related to reading) and to consider the possible neural mechanisms that might underlie these symptoms. Recent research has suggested that phonological difficulties may be just one piece, albeit a central one, in the jigsaw puzzle.

There is considerable heterogeneity in the skills of dyslexic children (inevitably given the very large numbers involved), but arguably the best cognitive level description of the general type of performance difficulty is that dyslexic children have difficulties when required to undertake fast, fluent, overlearned skills, or novel skills that involve the blending of two actions. Naturally this description applies in the literacy domain, with lack of automaticity in reading often cited as one of the key problems (Stanovich, 1988), and with evidence that dyslexic children require twice as long tachistoscopic presentation of a word as children matched for reading age (Yap and Vanderleij, 1993). It also seems to hold, at least for subgroups of dyslexic children, in cognitive non-literacy skills such as mathematics (Ackerman and Dykman, 1995), in general speed of information processing (Denckla and Rudel, 1976; Nicolson and Fawcett, 1994; Wolf and Bowers, 1999), and even in motor skills (Rudel, 1985; Wolff et al., 1990; Fawcett and Nicolson, 1995a).

In the light of the establishment of a wider range of difficulties, it is not surprising that two major recent theories expand significantly on the phonological deficit hypothesis. The double deficit hypothesis (Wolf and Bowers, 1999) suggests that dyslexia may arise from a deficit not only in phonological processing but also in terms of speed of processing. The magnocellular deficit hypotheses propose that the problems are attributable to abnormal sensory processing in the auditory (Tallal et al., 1993) or visual magnocellular pathways (e.g., Eden et al., 1996; Stein and Walsh, 1997).

There is no scope within this paper to consider further the above hypotheses here. A valuable recent overview is provided in (Demonet et al., 2004) and a wide-ranging account centred on phonological deficits is given in (Vellutino et al., 2004). In this article we present a further alternative framework that may appear radically different from phonological processing in that it focuses on learning rather than language, and on sub-cortical rather than cortical brain structures. Nonetheless, we see the framework as complementing rather than competing with phonological deficit – retaining speech and phonology at its core, but being broader and yet more specific. The framework has developed over the years, as we discovered more and more pieces of the jigsaw. The trail has led us from cognitive psychology to cognitive neuroscience to developmental science, but we believe that we now have a coherent account of the major symptoms, the underlying cause and the way the reading problems develop. Whether our account proves to be a complete explanation, or whether there are other important contributory causes, remain topics for further research, but on current evidence we consider the case cogent and compelling. For clarity we start at the beginning, and walk down the years.

The background

In our original research (Nicolson and Fawcett, 1990) we noted that, unlike language, reading is not a 'special' skill for humans. Humans are not evolutionarily adapted to read – few people could read at all until the last two or three hundred years. Consequently, in investigating why dyslexic children fail to learn to read, we felt an analysis of the learning processes involved must be of value. One of the critical aspects of learning a skill is to make it automatic, so that one can do it fluently without thinking about it. By adulthood, most skills – walking, talking, reading – are so deeply overlearned that we no longer have any insight into how we acquired them and consequently, to illustrate the processes involved, cognitive psychologists use two skills that are acquired relatively late in life. The skills involved are driving (which most adults eventually master pretty comprehensively) and typing (which most adults comprehensively fail to master). In learning to drive, the beginner can either steer, or change gear, but not both at the same time, because of the need to consciously attend to each procedure. An expert driver changes gear and steers 'automatically', thus leaving more 'capacity' for watching the traffic, planning a manoeuvre, or holding a conversation. Most of us when typing still have to look at the keyboard (even if using several fingers), and, compared with a touch-typist, our typing is slower, more error-prone and requires much more effort.

There is no theoretical reason to expect that automatisation of the processes in reading is qualitatively different from the general processes of automatising any other complex skill. Of course, automatisation is a key requirement for reading, and as noted above, there is extensive evidence that dyslexic children, even when reading well, are less fluent, requiring more time and effort to read than would a non-dyslexic child of the same reading age. Consequently we proposed the hypothesis that dyslexic children would have difficulty in automatising any skill (cognitive or motor). All dyslexia hypotheses predict poor reading and therefore critical tests of the hypothesis needed to be undertaken outside the reading domain. The automatisation deficit hypothesis was clearly supported by a set of experiments in which we asked dyslexic children to do two things at once. If a skill is automatic, then one ought to be able to do something else at the same time (assuming it does not directly interfere with

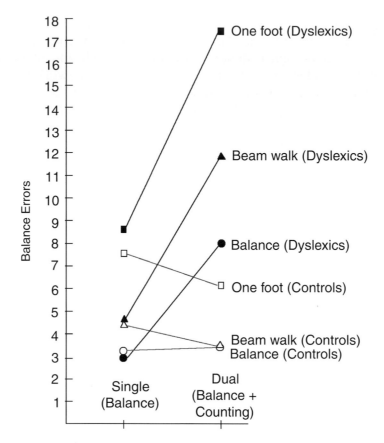

Fig. 1. Balance ability of dyslexic and control children under single- and dual-task conditions. Data redrawn from Nicolson and Fawcett (1990)

the first skill) with little or no loss of performance. A theoretically significant finding was for balance – a highly automatic skill with no language component. We found (Nicolson and Fawcett, 1990) that although a group of dyslexic adolescents[1] were normally able to balance as well as 'controls' (non-dyslexic children matched for age and IQ), their balance deteriorated very significantly when they had to do something else at the same time, whereas the controls' balance was not affected at all (Fig. 1). The deficit obtained for a range of secondary tasks, including concurrent counting, concurrent reaction time tasks, and blindfold balance (Fawcett and Nicolson, 1992). These findings strongly suggested that dyslexic children were not automatic even at the fundamental skill of balance. For some reason, dyslexic children had difficulty automatising skills, and had therefore to concentrate harder to achieve normal levels of

---

[1] In this, and all our subsequent studies, the proposal had been reviewed by the appropriate ethics committee, and the studies were performed in accordance with the ethical standards laid down in the 1964 Declaration of Helsinki. All persons gave their informed consent prior to participation. The criterion used for dyslexia was an IQ of 90 or more with reading age at least 18 months behind chronological age. In all studies after this 1990 study all dyslexic participants were explicitly screened for ADHD. Those showing clinically comorbid dyslexia and ADHD were excluded

performance. We have used the analogy of driving in a foreign country – one can do it, but it requires continual effort and is stressful and tiring over long periods. On our account, life for a dyslexic child is like always living in a foreign country. Alternatively, from the viewpoint of a dyslexic child, it may be as though the rest of the world touch types, whereas he or she has to look at the keyboard!

It may be valuable to report briefly two further extended studies that clarified the breadth of deficit and the locus of the deficit within the learning process.

Skill tests

In an attempt to minimise confounding factors arising from differences in experience together with use of compensatory strategies, we decided to test 'primitive' skills in the major modalities – skills that are not normally trained explicitly, and are not easily subject to compensatory strategies. In addition to psychometric tests, four types of test were used, namely tests of phonological skill, working memory, information processing speed, and motor skill (Fawcett and Nicolson, 1994, 1995a, b). In almost all tests of naming speed, phonological skill, motor skill, and also nonword repetition and articulation rate, the dyslexic children performed significantly worse than their chronological age controls. In general, the performance of the dyslexic children was somewhat below that of their reading age controls, but significant differences compared with reading age controls were obtained only for simple reaction (better performance than the reading age controls) and phonological skills, picture naming speed, bead threading and balance under dual task conditions or when blindfolded (worse than reading age controls).

Learning and dyslexia

One of the most severe limitations of the above work (and, indeed, of almost all dyslexia research) is that the investigations involve a 'snapshot' of the abilities of various groups of children at one point in time. For a sensitive analysis it is crucial to follow a child's performance over a period of time, while he or she acquires a skill. In the above skills tests we had established that the dyslexic children had normal speed of simple reaction (SRT). However, when a choice needed to be made, the dyslexic children were differentially affected by the increase in task complexity (Nicolson and Fawcett, 1994). We therefore undertook (Nicolson and Fawcett, 2000) a study investigating the time course of the blending of two separate simple reactions into a choice reaction (CRT).

In order to avoid any problems of left–right confusions or of stimulus discriminability, we used two stimuli of different modalities (tone and flash) and different effectors (hand and foot) for the two stimuli. Twenty-two subjects participated, 11 dyslexic and 11 control matched for age and IQ. In brief, following baseline performance monitoring on simple reaction to each stimulus separately, the two simple reaction tasks were combined into a choice reaction task in which half the stimuli were tones and half flashes, and the subject had to press the corresponding button, using the mapping established in the simple

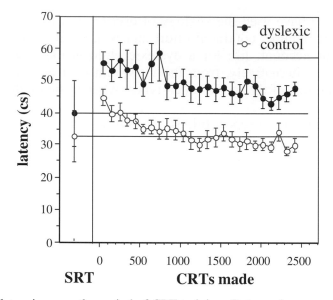

Fig. 2. Median latencies over the period of CRT training. Data are here averaged across hand and foot per participant and also across tone and flash. Data redrawn from Nicolson and Fawcett (2000)

reactions. Each session comprised three runs, each of 100 stimuli, and subjects kept returning every fortnight or so until their performance stopped improving (in terms of speed and accuracy). The results are shown in Fig. 2.

Analysis of the SRT performance indicated that there were no significant differences between the groups either for foot or hand, tone or flash. By contrast, initial performance on the CRT was significantly slower, and final performance was both significantly slower and less accurate for the dyslexic children. Initially the dyslexic group made slightly (but not significantly) more errors (13.8% vs 10.6%), indicating that the initial deficit cannot be attributable to some speed-accuracy trade-off by one group of children. However, by the final session the dyslexic group made around twice as many errors on average (9.1% vs 4.6%). Average learning rate for latency and accuracy was lower, but not significantly so, for the dyslexic group. Final choice reaction performance was very significantly both slower and less accurate than that of the controls both for hand and foot responses. Comparison of final hand and foot latency with the initial baseline SRT performance led to a dissociation, with both groups having significantly shorter final CRT latency than SRT latency for the foot responses, whereas for the hand responses the control group had equivalent latencies and the dyslexic group had significantly longer final CRT than SRT latencies.

The group data were then fitted using the appropriate 'power law' parametric technique (Newell and Rosenbloom, 1981). In brief, the curve fitted is $P(n) = A + Bn^{-\alpha}$ where $P(n)$ refers to performance on trial n, A is the asymptotic performance as n tends to infinity (taken as 0 here), B is a scaling parameter linked directly to initial performance, and α is the learning rate. The best fit curves for hand response CRT were $t = 53.9\ n^{-0.073}$ for the dyslexic children and $t = 39.4\ n^{-0.141}$ for the controls. For the foot responses the corresponding best fit curves were $t = 62.3\ n^{-0.086}$; $t = 50.4\ n^{-0.116}$ respectively. The parameter B was higher for the dyslexic children than the controls (around 30% on average), reflecting the slower initial performance on the CRT. The learning rate, α was about 1.5 times faster for the controls than the dyslexic children (0.141 vs. 0.073; 0.116 vs. 0.086 for the hand and foot responses respectively). This is a huge difference. Bearing in mind that the learning varies as a function of the time to the power α, if a skill takes a normal child 100 repetitions to master, it would take a dyslexic child $100^{1.5}$ i.e. 1,000 repetitions (10 times as long) to learn the skill to the same criterion, That is, their deficit increases with the square root of the time needed to learn the skill – our 'square root law'.

In summary, the dyslexic children appeared to have greater difficulty in blending existing skills into a new skill, and their performance after extensive practice (such that the skill was no longer improving noticeably) was slower and more error-prone. In other words, they were simply less skilled, their 'quality' of automatised performance was lower. It seems reasonable, therefore, to argue that this group of dyslexic children have difficulties both with the initial proceduralisation of skill, and with the 'quality' of skill post-training.

Taking these findings together, it is clear that automatisation deficit gives a good approximation to the range of difficulties suffered on a range of tasks, and captures reasonably well the general performance characteristics (lack of fluency, greater effort, more errors) established by 'snapshot' studies. Perhaps most satisfying, the hypothesis had ecological validity in that many dyslexic people and dyslexia practitioners came to us to say that our account seemed exactly right to them – they did have to concentrate on even the simplest skills.

On the other hand, what was not clear was why dyslexic children have problems in skill automatisation, and until this puzzle has been solved, the explanation was clearly incomplete. In the framework of (Morton and Frith, 1995) the automatisation deficit account (in common with the phonological deficit account and the double deficit account) provide an explanation at the cognitive level. The underlying cause(s) at the biological level were unspecified (and unclear).

In considering what might underlie the difficulties in automatisation, there is longstanding evidence of cerebellar involvement in automatisation: "*It is therefore suggested that the message sent down by the fore-brain in initiating a voluntary movement is often insufficient . . .: it needs to be further elaborated by the cerebellum in a manner that the cerebellum learns with practice, and this further elaboration makes use of information from sense organs. The cerebellum is thus a principal agent in the learning of motor skills*" (Brindley, 1964). For many years, Levinson (e.g., Frank and Levinson, 1973; Levinson, 1988) has argued that a vestibular impairment underlies the reading problems of dyslexic children. The vestibular system provides a major input to the cerebellum. However, vestibular impairment was discounted in mainstream dyslexia research because of the cerebellum's supposed lack of involvement in cognitive skill.

Around ten years ago, a complete re-evaluation of the role of the cerebellum in language processing was initiated as a result primarily of the revolution in brain imaging (facilitated by improved technology that allowed the whole brain to be imaged). It became clear that the cerebellum was highly active in a range of skills – when imagining a tennis stroke, when speaking, or even when trying to keep a list of words in memory. This apparent involvement of the cerebellum in cognitive skills led to considerable controversy in the field, in that the cerebellum had traditionally been considered as a motor area (Holmes, 1917, 1939; Eccles et al., 1967; Stein and Glickstein, 1992). However, as Leiner et al. (1989) noted, the human cerebellum (in particular, the lateral cerebellar hemispheres and ventrolateral cerebellar dentate nucleus) has evolved enormously, becoming linked not only with the frontal motor areas, but also some areas further forward in the frontal cortex, including Broca's language area. Leiner and his colleagues (Leiner et al., 1989, 1991, 1993) concluded that the cerebellum is therefore central for the acquisition of 'language dexterity'. In effect, then, they proposed that the cerebellum is critically involved in the automatisation of any skill, whether motor or cognitive.

When we originally put forward the cerebellar deficit hypotheses, the role of the cerebellum in cognition remained a controversial issue. Although there remains controversy over the role of the cerebellum in cognitive skills not involving speech or 'inner speech' (Glickstein, 1993; Ackermann et al., 1998), there is now general acceptance of the importance of the cerebellum in cognitive skills involving language (Ackermann and Hertrich, 2000; Fabbro et al., 2000; Silveri and Misciagna, 2000; Justus and Ivry, 2001; Marien et al., 2001). Of particular significance in the context of dyslexia are the recent findings of specific cerebellar activation in reading (Fulbright et al., 1999; Turkeltaub et al., 2002) and in verbal working memory (see Desmond and Fiez, 1998 for a review).

Putting together the then emerging 'cognitive neuroscience' results on the role of the cerebellum in skill automatisation, balance and language dexterity with our own findings with dyslexic children, it seemed evident that cerebellar abnormality was a prime candidate for the cause of the difficulties suffered by dyslexic children (Nicolson et al., 1995).

The cerebellum

The cerebellum is a very densely packed and deeply folded subcortical brain structure situated at the back of the brain, sometimes known as the 'hind-brain' (Holmes, 1939). In humans, it accounts for 10–15% of brain weight, 40% of brain surface area, and 50% of the brain's neurons, with 10^{11} granule cells alone (Brodal, 1981). There are two cerebellar hemispheres, each comprising folded cerebellar cortex, which receive massive inputs from all the senses, from the primary motor cortex, and from many other areas of cerebral cortex, either by 'mossy fibres' from the pontine nuclei or via 'climbing fibres' from the inferior olive. Output from the cerebellum is generated by Purkinje cells, goes via the deep cerebellar nuclei (dentate, interposed and fastigial nuclei), and is generally inhibitory. The cerebellar cortex comprises several phylogenetically ancient structures, including the flocculonodular node, which is situated at the caudal end, and receives input from the vestibular system and projects to the vestibular nuclei. The vermis, located on the midline, receives visual, auditory, cutaneous and kinesthetic information from sensory nuclei, and sends output to the fastigial nucleus, which connects to the vestibular nucleus and motor neurons in the reticular formation. On both sides of the vermis, the intermediate zone receives input from the motor areas of cerebral cortex through the pontine tegmental reticular nucleus. Output is via the interposed nucleus, which projects to the red nucleus, and thence the rubrospinal system for arm and hand movements, and also to the ventrothalamic nucleus.

The lateral zone of the cerebellum is phylogenetically more recent, and is much larger in humans (relative to overall brain size) than in other primates (Passingham, 1975) and is referred to as the neocerebellum. It is involved in the control of independent limb movements and especially in rapid, skilled movements, receiving information from frontal association cortex and from primary motor cortex via the pontine nucleus. It also receives somatosensory information about the current position and rate of movement of the limbs. Its role in skilled movement execution is generally thought to be the computation of the appropriate movement parameters for the next movement (possibly the next but one movement), and to communicate these via the dentate nucleus and the ventrolateral thalamic nucleus to the primary motor cortex. The lateral zone also sends outputs to the red nucleus, and thus the rubrospinal tract. The cerebellum is one of the first brain structures to begin to differentiate, arising from two different germinal matrices, yet it is one of the last to achieve maturity – the cellular organization of the cerebellum continues to change for many months after birth. This protracted developmental process creates a special susceptibility to disruptions during embryogenesis (Wang and Zoghbi, 2001).

Damage to different parts of the cerebellum can lead to different symptoms. In humans, damage to the flocculonodular system or vermis may typically lead to disturbances in posture and balance. Damage to the intermediate zone causes problems such as limb rigidity in the rubrospinal system. Damage to the lateral zone causes weakness (loss of muscle tone) and dyscoordination or decomposition of movement (that is, previously coordinated sequences of movements, such as picking up a cup, may break down into a series of separate movements). Lesions of the lateral zone also appear to impair the timing of rapid ballistic (pre-planned, automatic) movements. However, one of the features of cerebellar damage is the great plasticity of the system. Typically normal or close to normal performance is attained again within a few months of the initial damage (Holmes, 1922).

One of the fascinating aspects of the cerebellum is that the structure of the cerebellum appears to be quite different from that of the rest of the brain. In particular, the cerebellar cortex comprises a mosaic of relatively independent 'microzones', comprising a Purkinje cell and its associated inputs and output. These microzones, in combination with the associated pathways to and from the associated extra-cerebellar nuclei, may be thought of as a 'cerebellar-cortico-nuclear microcomplex' (CCMC) able to undertake a range of tasks (Ito, 1984). Many models have been proposed for cerebellar function, but the Marr/Albus composite model (Marr, 1969; Albus, 1971), in which the climbing fibres act as an error signal to the CCMC, remains a good approximation both for skill acquisition and execution (Thach, 1996).

Recall Brindley's insight that the cerebellum might be used like a co-processor to calculate the necessary muscle-level details to effect a high level cortical command. In this context, a particularly interesting observation is that of (Ito, 1990), who noted that many skills could be construed as developing from a *feedback* model (in which a movement is made under conscious control, and the match between say hand and target is monitored continually), to a *feedforward* model ('if I send these instructions to my hand it will end up at position *P* at time *t*') to an *inverse* model ('in order to touch the button, I need to execute the following [set of actions]'). An inverse model would therefore allow the cerebral cortex to send the command 'touch the button', downloading the calculations to the cerebellum. Ito makes it clear that the CCMC provides the appropriate learning and monitoring equipment to achieve these learning changes from voluntary to automatic movements, and goes on to speculate that a very similar set of cerebellum-based procedures could be used to acquire more and more practised cognitive skills. He outlined a physiologically-inspired model of how this could be achieved in the case of the vestibulo-ocular reflex (VOR) – keeping an image steady on the retina when moving the head. This was taken further by (Kawato and Gomi, 1992), with their feedback error learning algorithm. Recently, Dean et al. (2002) provide an alternative neuro-physiologically plausible 'decorrelation control' algorithm, modelled on cerebellar circuitry, able to learn to achieve the necessary compensation for the inertia etc. of the oculomotor system in the VOR.

Evaluations of the cerebellar deficit in dyslexia

Over the past decade we have completed a series of investigations of the cerebellar deficit hypothesis. The initial study replicated (Ivry and Keele, 1989) who claimed that the cerebellum was involved in timing functions based on their finding that cerebellar patients had a specific deficit in time estimation but not in loudness estimation. The replication (Nicolson et al., 1995) established that the same pattern of intact loudness estimation and markedly impaired time estimation also characterised our dyslexic panel.

The classic signs of damage to the cerebellum (Holmes, 1917; Dow and Moruzzi, 1958) are dysmetria (difficulty in precisely measured movements) and dystonia (low muscle tone). Consequently, we administered clinical tests of cerebellar dysfunction on our panel of dyslexic and control children (Fawcett et al., 1996). We established that the dyslexic children showed marked deficits on almost all of these clinical tests, and we then replicated these findings on further populations of dyslexic and control children, establishing that around 80% of our sample of 80 dyslexic children showed clear 'cerebellar' symptoms[2] (Fawcett and Nicolson, 1999). These findings were completely unexpected from the literature and were not predicted from any other theory of dyslexia, and consequently they provided strong support for the hypothesis. Nonetheless,

---

[2] One of the major difficulties in investigating and interpreting cerebellar signs is that of establishing objective, robust and specific tests of cerebellar function. This reflects the extensive linkage of the cerebellum to sensory, motor and cognitive areas, its plasticity, and its involvement in acquisition and execution. We consider that the establishment of better and more specific tests of cerebellar function is a critical task for cognitive neuroscience

it could still be argued that it was not the cerebellum itself, but perhaps some input to, or output from, the cerebellum that was causing the problems. This is by no means an unlikely hypothesis because the cerebellum has two way connections with almost all parts of the brain, including the language areas, and also of course receives input from sensory and vestibular pathways.

The above tests of cerebellar function were necessarily indirect. In considering the design of a direct test, we wished to undertake a functional imaging study, but, rather than select one in the reading-related domain (for which differences in performance – and possibly anxiety – cloud interpretation of imaging data) we preferred to study a task outside the literacy domain in which there was clear evidence of strong cerebellar activation in normal subjects. Fortunately, a PET study (Jenkins et al., 1994) provided a perfect opportunity. Jenkins and his colleagues had their subjects learn a sequence of 8 button presses by trial and error using a 4-key response board with one key per finger. They established clear increases in cerebellar activation (compared with rest) both when the subjects were executing a previously overlearned (automatic) sequence of presses and also when they were learning a new sequence of presses. We undertook a precise replication, using the oldest members (now adult) of our dyslexic and control panels. Compared with the controls, the dyslexic participants showed significantly less cerebellar activation in the ipsilateral (right) posterior lobe of the cerebellum. Interestingly, similar results obtained for both tasks – executing the previously overlearned sequence, and learning the new sequence. Overall the dyslexic group showed barely any increase in activation in the right cerebellar hemisphere and vermis (around 10% of that of the controls). This suggests strongly that, unlike non-dyslexic adults, dyslexic adults do not activate the cerebellum in these learning and automatic tasks – presumably because it does not help them in the normal way. This PET study therefore confirmed that the behavioural cerebellar signs of these subjects did indeed reflect abnormal cerebellar function, and therefore lent weight to the above behavioural studies.

Consequently, at least for the dyslexic children in our panel, we have found both behavioural and neurological evidence of cerebellar abnormality, thereby providing strong support for cerebellar deficit hypothesis.

Finally, arguably the most direct, and certainly the most intriguing, evidence of abnormality in dyslexia derives from the collection of dyslexic and non-dyslexic brains in the Beth Israel/International Dyslexia Association Brain Bank (Boston, USA), which was established by Norman Geschwind. Early work (e.g., Galaburda et al., 1985) revealed microscopical abnormalities in the dyslexic brains, with subsequent work indicating that there were also abnormalities in the magnocellular pathways from eye and ear (Galaburda and Livingstone, 1993; Galaburda et al., 1994). In a neuroanatomical investigation of the cerebellar regions of these specimens, using a blind analysis procedure Finch established significant abnormality (Finch et al., 2002), characterised by greater cell size, in both the cerebellum and in the inferior olive (a nucleus in the brain stem that sends input to the cerebellum). Interestingly, the effect size of these abnormalities was even greater than that established for the magnocellular pathways (Livingstone et al., 1991).

Converging direct evidence of cerebellar dysfunction is also provided by a study (Rae et al., 1998) of metabolic abnormalities in dyslexic men. Rae and her colleagues obtained localised proton magnetic resonance spectra bilaterally from the temporo-parietal cortex and cerebellum of 14 dyslexic men and 15 control men of similar age. Bilateral MR spectroscopy indicated significant differences in the ratio of choline containing compounds to N-acetylaspartate (NA) in the left temporo-parietal lobe and the right cerebellum, together with lateralisation differences in the cerebellum of the dyslexic men but not the controls. The authors concluded (p. 1849) that *"These differences provide direct evidence of the involvement of the cerebellum in dyslexic dysfunction"*. Further evidence of anatomical cerebellar differences in dyslexic subjects is reported by (Rae et al., 2002) who found greater cerebellar symmetry in dyslexia, with degree of symmetry correlating with degree of phonological deficit. (Leonard, 2001) report marked leftward asymmetry of the anterior lobe of the cerebellum as one of four markers for dyslexia. (Brown et al., 2001) report evidence of decreases in gray matter in dyslexic subjects, most notably in the left temporal lobe and bilaterally in the temporo-parieto-occipital juncture, but also in the frontal lobe, caudate, thalamus, and cerebellum. A subsequent volumetric investigation (Eckert et al., 2003) established significant differences between matched dyslexic and control children related to cerebral volume, pars triangularis and anterior right cerebellum. Multivariate analyses of brain volume and behavioural data suggested a dissociation, with pars triangularis associated with phonology and rapid naming whereas the anterior cerebellum volume was associated with phonology, rapid naming and orthography. In short, while there is still not a complete convergence of data, there is now extensive evidence of structural differences in the cerebellum of dyslexic individuals.

The causal chain

This converging multidisciplinary evidence of cerebellar abnormality in dyslexia led us to develop an 'ontogenetic causal chain' analysis (Fig. 3) intended to address the issue of whether cerebellar dysfunction alone could be sufficient to account for the know specific difficulties of dyslexic children (the strong form of the hypothesis). It should be noted that investigation of this strong form in no way precludes the possibility that other brain areas might also be affected. We proposed in brief that cerebellar abnormality from birth leads to slight speech output dysfluency, then receptive speech problems (i.e., difficulties in analysing the speech sounds) and thence deficiencies in phonological awareness (Nicolson et al., 2001). Taken together with the problems in skill automatisation and coordination associated with the cerebellar impairment, this analysis provides not only a good account of the pattern of difficulties suffered by dyslexic children, but also how they arise developmentally. This causal chain analysis still awaits evaluation via studies of pre-school 'dyslexic' children, but if supported by further research, it provides a significant demonstration of how abnormality in a brain structure (the cerebellum) can lead, via difficulties in cognitive processes such as automatisation and phonology, to deficits in arguably the pinnacle of cognitive skill, namely reading.

Dyslexia: An ontogenetic causal chain

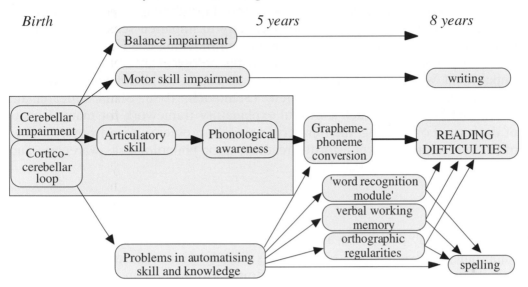

Fig. 3. A hypothetical causal chain. The horizontal axis represents both the passage of time (experience) and also the ways that difficulties with skill acquisition cause subsequent problems, leading to the known difficulties in reading, writing and spelling. The text provides a fuller explanation of the processes involved. Of particular interest is the progression highlighted as a central feature. Cerebellar abnormality at birth leads to mild motor and articulatory problems. Lack of articulatory fluency leads in turn to an impoverished representation of the phonological characteristics of speech, and thence to the well-established difficulties in phonological awareness at around 5 years that lead to subsequent problems in learning to read. Other routes outline the likely problems outside the phonological domain, and indicate that the difficulties in learning to read, spell and write may derive from a number of inter-dependent factors

Note that the three criterial difficulties in the World Federation of Neurology definition – writing, reading and spelling – are all accounted for in different ways. It may be useful to distinguish between direct and indirect cerebellar causation. Cerebellar deficit provides a natural, direct, explanation of the poor quality of handwriting frequently shown by dyslexic children (Martlew, 1992). Handwriting, of course, is a motor skill that requires precise timing and co-ordination of diverse muscle groups. Literacy difficulties arise from several routes. The central route is highlighted. If an infant has a cerebellar impairment, initial direct manifestations will include a mild motor difficulty – the infant may be slower to sit up and to walk – and crucially, the direct effect on articulation would suggest that the infant might be slower to start babbling (see e.g., Davis and MacNeilage, 2000; Ejiri and Masataka, 2001; MacNeilage and Davis, 2001), and, later, talking (cf. Green et al., 2000; Bates and Dick, 2002). Even after speech and walking emerge, one might expect that the skills would be less fluent, less 'dextrous', in infants with cerebellar impairment. If articulation is less fluent than normal, then one indirect effect is that it takes up more conscious resources, leaving fewer resources to process the ensuing sensory feedback. An additional indirect effect is that reduced articulation speed leads to reduced effective 'working memory' as reflected in the 'phonological loop' (Baddeley et al., 1975). This, in turn leads to difficulties in language acquisition (Gathercole and Baddeley, 1989). Furthermore, reduced quality of articulatory representation might lead directly to impaired sensitivity to onset, rime, and the phonemic structure of language (Snowling and Hulme, 1994) – in short, one would expect early deficits in phonological awareness. Cerebellar impairment would therefore be predicted to cause, by direct and by indirect means, the 'phonological core deficit' (Stanovich, 1988; Shankweiler et al., 1995) that has proved such a fruitful explanatory framework for many aspects of dyslexia. For spelling, the third criterial skill, problems arise from a number of indirect routes – over-effortful reading, poor phonological awareness, and difficulties in automatising skills.

Conclusions

We conclude by noting that the cerebellar deficit framework has a number of important positive features. First, it links directly with 'mainstream' theories in cognitive psychology (learning and automatisation) and in cognitive neuro-science (speech-based cognition and the cerebellum). This provides a natural channel for progress and cross-fertilisation in both directions. Second, the explicit representation both of a 'biological' level of analysis (cerebellum) and a 'cognitive' level of analysis (automaticity and learning) provides an important link to genetics in one direction and education and treatment in the other. Third, the 'ontogenetic' approach, which asks how the reading problems develop as a function of brain characteristics and experience (see also Lyytinen et al., 2001), facilitates the development of diagnostic techniques that can be undertaken before a dyslexic child starts (and fails) to learn to read (cf. Nicolson and Fawcett, 1996) and also provides potentially fruitful theoretical justifications for pre-school support methods.

We should emphasise, however, that, despite the above desirable features, the cerebellar deficit hypothesis should be seen as incompletely proven at this stage, in that the dyslexia-related data provided are mostly from small scale studies in our own laboratory. The approach raises many further theoretical questions: are there sub-types of dyslexia corresponding to different loci of abnormality in the cerebellum; to what extent do cerebellar and magnocellular deficits co-occur; how do these specific issues relate to underlying genetic endowment; are there other developmental disorders that might also correspond to cerebellar impairment; is it possible to move toward diagnostic principles for developmental disability inspired by brain-based investigation rather than behaviour-based classification; above all, how can knowledge of underlying causality inform support and remediation? These are all potentially fruitful research issues, and we consider their investigation will continue to illuminate the complex interplay between the brain, the environment and behaviour, in both normal and abnormal development.

Above all, we hope that the ecosystem (Nicolson, 2002) of policy makers, researchers practitioners and people with dyslexia – whatever their perspec-tive – will combine to enhance, modify and transform the theoretical views expressed here (and by other approaches) so as to encompass the full range of potential causative factors, leading to a unified framework that integrates theory, diagnosis and support for children with dyslexia.

References

Ackerman PT, Dykman RA (1995) Reading-disabled students with and without comorbid arithmetic disability. Dev Neuropsychol 11: 351–371

Ackermann H, Hertrich I (2000) The contribution of the cerebellum to speech processing. J Neurolinguist 13: 95–116

Ackermann H, Wildgruber D, Daum I, Grodd W (1998) Does the cerebellum contribute to cognitive aspects of speech production? A functional magnetic resonance imaging (fMRI) study in humans. Neurosci Lett 247: 187–190

Albus JS (1971) A theory of cerebellar function. Math Biosci 10: 25–61

Baddeley AD, Thomson N, Buchanan M (1975) Word length and the structure of short term memory. J Verbal Learn Verbal Behav 14: 575–589

Badian NA (1984) Reading disability in an epidemiological context: incidence and environmental correlates. J Learn Disabil 17: 129–136

Bates E, Dick F (2002) Language, gesture, and the developing brain. Dev Psychobiol 40: 293–310

Bradley L, Bryant PE (1983) Categorising sounds and learning to read: a causal connection. Nature 301: 419–421

Brindley GS (1964) The use made by the cerebellum of the information that it receives from the sense organs. Int Brain Res Org Bull 3: 80

Brodal A (1981) The cerebellum. In: Brodal A (ed) Neurological anatomy in relation to clinical medicine. Oxford University Press, Oxford, pp 294–393

Brown WE, Eliez S, Menon V, Rumsey JM, White CD, Reiss AL (2001) Preliminary evidence of widespread morphological variations of the brain in dyslexia. Neurology 56: 781–783

Davis BL, MacNeilage PF (2000) An embodiment perspective on the acquisition of speech perception. Phonetica 57: 229–241

Dean P, Porrill J, Stone JV (2002) Decorrelation control by the cerebellum achieves oculomotor plant compensation in simulated vestibulo-ocular refelx. Proc Roy Soc Lond B 269: 1895–1904

Demonet JF, Taylor MJ, Chaix Y (2004) Developmental dyslexia. Lancet 363: 1451–1460

Denckla MB, Rudel RG (1976) Rapid 'Automatized' naming (R.A.N.). Dyslexia differentiated from other learning disabilities. Neuropsychologia 14: 471–479

Dow RS, Moruzzi G (1958) The physiology and pathology of the cerebellum. University of Minnesota Press, Minneapolis

Eccles JC, Ito M, Szentagothai J (1967) The cerebellum as a neuronal machine. Springer, New York

Eckert MA, Leonard CM, Richards TL, Aylward EH, Thomson J, Berninger VW (2003) Anatomical correlates of dyslexia: frontal and cerebellar findings. Brain 126: 482–494

Eden GF, VanMeter JW, Rumsey JM, Maisog JM, Woods RP, Zeffiro TA (1996) Abnormal processing of visual motion in dyslexia revealed by functional brain imaging. Nature 382: 66–69

Ejiri K, Masataka N (2001) Co-occurrence of preverbal vocal behavior and motor action in early infancy. Dev Sci 4: 40–48

Fabbro F, Moretti R, Bava A (2000) Language impairments in patients with cerebellar lesions. J Neurolinguist 13: 173–188

Fawcett AJ, Nicolson RI (1992) Automatisation deficits in balance for dyslexic children. Percept Mot Skills 75: 507–529

Fawcett AJ, Nicolson RI (1994) Naming speed in children with dyslexia. J Learning Disabil 27: 641–646

Fawcett AJ, Nicolson RI (1995a) Persistent deficits in motor skill for children with dyslexia. J Motor Behav 27: 235–241

Fawcett AJ, Nicolson RI (1995b) Persistence of phonological awareness deficits in older children with dyslexia. Reading and Writing 7: 361–376

Fawcett AJ, Nicolson RI (1999) Performance of dyslexic children on cerebellar and cognitive tests. J Motor Behav 31: 68–78

Fawcett AJ, Nicolson RI, Dean P (1996) Impaired performance of children with dyslexia on a range of cerebellar tasks. Ann Dyslexia 46: 259–283

Finch AJ, Nicolson RI, Fawcett AJ (2002) Evidence for a neuroanatomical difference within the olivo-cerebellar pathway of adults with dyslexia. Cortex 38: 529–539

Frank J, Levinson HN (1973) Dysmetric dyslexia and dyspraxia: hypothesis and study. J Am Acad Child Psychiatry 12: 690–701

Fulbright RK, Jenner AR, Mencl WE, Pugh KR, Shaywitz BA, Shaywitz SE, Frost SJ, Skudlarski P, Constable RT, Lacadie CM, Marchione KE, Gore JC (1999) The cerebellum's role in reading: a functional MR imaging study. Am J Neuroradiol 20: 1925–1930

Galaburda A, Livingstone M (1993) Evidence for a magnocellular defect in developmental dyslexia. Ann NY Acad Sci 682: 70–82

Galaburda AM, Sherman GF, Rosen GD, Aboitiz F, Geschwind N (1985) Developmental dyslexia – 4 consecutive patients with cortical anomalies. Ann Neurol 18: 222–233

Galaburda AM, Menard MT, Rosen GD (1994) Evidence for aberrant auditory anatomy in developmental dyslexia. Proc Natl Acad Sci USA 91: 8010–8013

Gathercole SE, Baddeley AD (1989) Evaluation of the role of phonological STM in the development of vocabulary in children: a longitudinal study. J Memory Language 28: 200–213

Glickstein M (1993) Motor skills but not cognitive tasks. Trends Neurosci 16: 450–451

Green JR, Moore CA, Higashikawa M, Steeve RW (2000) The physiologic development of speech motor control: lip and jaw coordination. J Speech Language Hearing Res 43: 239–255

Holmes G (1917) The symptoms of acute cerebellar injuries due to gunshot injuries. Brain 40: 461–535

Holmes G (1922) Clinical symptoms of cerebellar disease and their interpretation. Lancet 1: 1177–1237

Holmes G (1939) The cerebellum of man. Brain 62: 1–30

Ito M (1984) The cerebellum and neural control. Raven Press, New York

Ito M (1990) A new physiological concept on cerebellum. Rev Neurol (Paris) 146: 564–569

Ivry RB, Keele SW (1989) Timing functions of the cerebellum. J Cogn Neurosci 1: 136–152

Jenkins IH, Brooks DJ, Nixon PD, Frackowiak RSJ, Passingham RE (1994) Motor sequence learning – a study with Positron Emission Tomography. J Neurosci 14: 3775–3790

Jorm AF, Share DL, McLean R, Matthews D (1986) Cognitive factors at school entry predictive of specific reading retardation and general reading backwardness: a research note. J Child Psychol Psychiatry Allied Disciplines 27: 45–54

Justus TC, Ivry RB (2001) The cognitive neuropsychology of the cerebellum. Int Rev Psychiatry 13: 276–282

Kawato M, Gomi H (1992) The cerebellum and VOR/OKR learning models. Trends Neurosci 15: 445–452

Leiner HC, Leiner AL, Dow RS (1989) Reappraising the cerebellum: what does the hindbrain contribute to the forebrain. Behav Neurosci 103: 998–1008

Leiner HC, Leiner AL, Dow RS (1991) The human cerebro-cerebellar system: its computing, cognitive, and language skills. Behav Brain Res 44: 113–128

Leiner HC, Leiner AL, Dow RS (1993) Cognitive and language functions of the human cerebellum. Trends Neurosci 16: 444–447

Leonard CM (2001) Imaging brain structure in children: differentiating language disability and reading disability. Learning Disabil Quart 24: 158–176

Levinson HN (1988) The cerebellar-vestibular basis of learning disabilities in children, adolescents and adults: hypothesis and study. Percept Mot Skills 67: 983–1006

Livingstone MS, Rosen GD, Drislane FW, Galaburda AM (1991) Physiological and anatomical evidence for a magnocellular defect in developmental dyslexia. Proc Natl Acad Sci USA 88: 7943–7947

Lyytinen H, Ahonen T, Eklund K, Guttorm TK, Laakso ML, Leinonen S, Leppanan PHT, Lyytinen P, Poikkeus AM, Puolakanaho A, Richardson U, Viholainen H (2001) Developmental pathways of children with and without familial risk for dyslexia during the first years of life. Dev Neuropsychol 20: 535–554

MacNeilage PF, Davis BL (2001) Motor mechanisms in speech ontogeny: phylogenetic, neurobiological and linguistic implications. Curr Opin Neurobiol 11: 696–700

Marien P, Engelborghs S, Fabbro F, De Deyn PP (2001) The lateralized linguistic cerebellum: a review and a new hypothesis. Brain Language 79: 580–600

Marr D (1969) A theory of cerebellar cortex. J Physiol (Lond) 202: 437–470

Martlew M (1992) Handwriting and spelling – dyslexic childrens abilities compared with children of the same chronological age and younger children of the same spelling level. Br J Educ Psychol 62: 375–390

Morton J, Frith U (1995) Causal modelling: a structural approach to developmental psychopathology. In: Cicchetti D (ed) Manual of developmental psychopathology. Wiley, New York, pp 274–298

Newell A, Rosenbloom PS (1981) Mechanisms of skill acquisition and the law of practice. In: Anderson JR (ed) Cognitive skills and their acquisition. Lawrence Erlbaum, Hillsdale, NJ

Nicolson RI (2002) The dyslexia ecosystem. Dyslexia: Int J Res Pract 8: 55–66

Nicolson RI, Fawcett AJ (1990) Automaticity: a new framework for dyslexia research? Cognition 35: 159–182

Nicolson RI, Fawcett AJ (1994) Reaction times and dyslexia. Quart J Exp Psychol 47A: 29–48

Nicolson RI, Fawcett AJ (1996) The dyslexia early screening test. The Psychological Corporation, London

Nicolson RI, Fawcett AJ (2000) Long-term learning in dyslexic children. Eur J Cogn Psychol 12: 357–393

Nicolson RI, Fawcett AJ, Dean P (1995) Time-estimation deficits in developmental dyslexia – evidence for cerebellar involvement. Proc Roy Soc Lond Series B-Biol Sci 259: 43–47

Nicolson RI, Fawcett AJ, Dean P (2001) Developmental dyslexia: the cerebellar deficit hypothesis. Trends Neurosci 24: 508–511

Passingham RE (1975) Changes in the size and organization of the brain in man and his ancestors. Brain Behav Evol 11: 73–90

Rae C, Lee MA, Dixon RM, Blamire AM, Thompson CH, Styles P, Talcott J, Richardson AJ, Stein JF (1998) Metabolic abnormalities in developmental dyslexia detected by H-1 magnetic resonance spectroscopy. Lancet 351: 1849–1852

Rae C, Harasty JA, Dzendrowskyj TE, Talcott JB, Simpson JM, Blamire AM, Dixon RM, Lee MA, Thompson CH, Styles P, Richardson AJ, Stein JF (2002) Cerebellar morphology in developmental dyslexia. Neuropsychologia 40: 1285–1292

Rudel RG (1985) The definition of dyslexia: language and motor deficits. In: Duffy FH, Geschwind N (eds) Dyslexia: a neuroscientific approach to clinical evaluation. Little Brown, Boston

Shankweiler D, Crain S, Katz L, Fowler AE, Liberman AM, Brady SA, Thornton R, Lundquist E, Dreyer L, Fletcher JM, Stuebing KK, Shaywitz SE, Shaywitz BA (1995) Cognitive profiles of reading-disabled children – comparison of language-skills in phonology, morphology, and syntax. Psychol Sci 6: 149–156

Silveri MC, Misciagna S (2000) Language, memory, and the cerebellum. J Neurolinguist 13: 129–143

Snowling M (1987) Dyslexia: a cognitive developmental perspective. Blackwell, Oxford

Snowling M, Hulme C (1994) The development of phonological skills. Phil Transact Roy Soc Lond Series B-Biol Sci 346: 21–27

Stanovich KE (1988) Explaining the differences between the dyslexic and the garden-variety poor reader: the phonological-core variable-difference model. J Learn Disabil 21: 590–604

Stein J, Walsh V (1997) The magnocellular deficit theory of dyslexia – reply. Trends Neurosci 20: 398

Stein JF, Glickstein M (1992) Role of the cerebellum in visual guidance of movement. Physiol Rev 72: 972–1017

Thach WT (1996) On the specific role of the cerebellum in motor learning and cognition: clues from PET activation and lesion studies in man. Behav Brain Sci 19: 411–431

Turkeltaub PE, Eden GF, Jones KM, Zeffiro TA (2002) Meta-analysis of the functional neuroanatomy of single-word reading: method and validation. Neuroimage 16: 765–780

Vellutino FR (1979) Dyslexia: theory and research. MIT Press, Cambridge

Vellutino FR, Fletcher JM, Snowling M, Scanlon DM (2004) Specific reading disability (dyslexia): what have we learned in the past four decades? J Child Psychol Psychiatry 45: 2–40

Wang VY, Zoghbi HY (2001) Genetic regulation of cerebellar development. Nature Rev Neurosci 2: 484–491

Wolf M, Bowers PG (1999) The double-deficit hypothesis for the developmental dyslexias. J Educ Psychol 91: 415–438

Wolff PH, Michel GF, Ovrut M (1990) Rate variables and automatized naming in developmental dyslexia. Brain Language 39: 556–575

World Federation of Neurology (1968) Report of research group on dyslexia and world illiteracy. WFN, Dallas

Yap R, Vanderleij A (1993) Word-processing in dyslexics – an automatic decoding deficit. Reading Writing 5: 261–27

Authors' address: Prof. R. Nicolson, Department of Psychology, University of Sheffield, Western Bank, Sheffield S10 2TP, United Kingdom, e-mail: r.nicolson@shef.ac.uk

Disorders of speech development: diagnostic and treatment aspects

P. G. Zorowka

Department for Hearing, Speech and Voice Disorders, Medical University,
Innsbruck, Austria

Summary. Language acquisition is a complex process relying on the well-tuned interaction of a variety of factors. Its genetic base is still little explored, but perhaps plays the most important role during the early periods of this process. In addition, neurological, cognitive and emotional abilities of the child as well as verbal stimulation from the environment are crucial.

Language development disorders manifest themselves as late onset, slow progression or as erroneous course of the language development. Because of the multitude of factors involved, their aetiology is frequently difficult to determine. Diagnosis of such disorders commonly requires the cooperation of several professionals, like paediatricians, otolaryngologists, psychologists, and speech pathologists.

The "late bloomer" hypothesis suggests, that up to 50% of children presenting with language problems in early years, make up for them without intervention up to age four years. Nevertheless, treatment for a language problem, as soon as it appears, is generally recommended in order to minimize adverse effects on succeeding developmental steps.

Introduction

Phylogenetically, speech is one of the most recent achievements in the evolution of the human species and it is perhaps also the most distinguished one. Without speech, or any sophisticated form of communication, human individuals and their societies are unable to exist or survive. From the very first breath, life and the development of the individual depend on successful communicative interaction with fellow human. And throughout life, an individual relies on his/her ability to express wishes or needs, to impart observations or experiences, to convey information or knowledge, and to understand these utterances when articulated by others. If not, integration into society would not be possible.

As human societies become more and more complex, the demands on the communicative abilities of their members grow. It is probably for this reason that disorders of speech development receive more attention today than ever

Table 1. Change in occupation from 1900 to 2000
(Ruben, 2000)

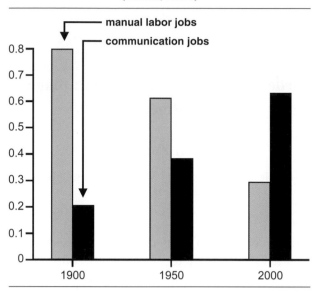

before in history (Table 1). The question whether they are more frequent today than in former decades or centuries is difficult to answer. As a matter of fact, a language disturbance is a serious handicap to social interaction in a world where 90% of all professions rely on communication in one form or another. (Table 2).

The devastating impact of impaired communication affects not only the social functioning, but above all the personality of the individual. As speech development goes hand in hand with cognitive development, a reduction in speech-mediated stimulation will cause reduced evolution of cognitive skills. The forming of personality characteristics like intelligence, attitudes towards values, or open-mindedness, is largely dependent on the ability to make fine conceptual differences – an ability essentially based on the availability of a powerful system of signs (called language). In this regard, language development

Table 2. Employment and unemployment rates and communication disorders

Condition	Affected persons (n)	% Employed	# Employed	% Unemployed	# Unemployed
Working age population with employment and without disab.	138,142,000	74.8	103,330,260	25.2	34,811,780
With non severe disability	16,497,000	74.1	12,224,277	25.9	4,272,723
With severe disability	14,392,000	25.5	3,669,960	74.5	10,722,040
Difficulty hearing	5,837,000	64.4	3,759,028	**35.6**	2,077,972
Unable to hear	430,000	50.4	216,700	**49.6**	213,280
Difficulty in speaking understandably	1,520,000	32.4	492,480	**67.6**	1,027,520
Unable to speak understandably	172,000	24.4	41,968	**75.6**	130,032
Total communication disorders	7,959,000	56.7	4,510,196	43.3	348,804

disorders – even in their minimal forms – may have sustainable adverse effects on the development of the affected individual.

Although the process of language acquisition continues throughout a person's entire life, there is general consensus that there are "critical periods" for speech development in infancy and early childhood. During these periods, the brain is best able to adopt a language and integrate it into the neuronal network that forms the basis for all behavioral and intellectual skills. At a later age, the effort to learn a language will be more difficult and perhaps less effective. Factors that interfere with language acquisition during this critical period – e.g. hearing impairment, mental retardation, or insufficient verbal stimulation from other persons – cause more substantial damage to the individual's language skills than do factors interfering at later ages.

Language acquisition starts long before an infant utters its first words. Some studies suggest that the process starts even before birth, because fetuses seem to already recognize the maternal voice and to respond to prosody patterns (Rosetti, 2001). Initial forms of communication occur when the newborn cries in order to obtain food, companionship, or comfort. A few months after birth the infant begins to realize that some sounds are important and distinctively reacts to them. By six months of age, most children recognize the basic sounds of their native language. Further preparatory steps take place between ages 6 and 12 months, where the ongoing maturation of expressive speech mechanisms (tongue, lips, jaw) enables the infant to produce controlled sounds. At this age, "babbling", the repetition of syllables, is considered to be a pre-verbal manifestation of normal speech development. By age 9 months, babbling turns into a type of nonsense speech, that includes modulated sounds as a new element. By age 1 year, most children manage to say a few words, commonly the names of family members. From this point on, the child begins to recognize that certain sounds have a meaning and that they can be used to make other people respond to them. Between age 1 and 2 years, children learn to understand simple requests and questions like "where is the cat?", and produce a "jargon" language or a mix of made-up words and understandable words. At age 18 months, they are able to say some ten words that are intelligible to family members. They also know the names of several body parts, people, and objects. By age 2 years, they start to combine words, and the initial two-word utterances soon give way to three- and four-word sentences. During the third year of life, the child learns the meaning of some spatial concepts ("in", "on") and of pronouns ("me", "you"). Speech becomes more accurate, but may still leave off ending sounds, so that strangers are not able to understand much of what is said. Towards the end of the third year, the toddlers begin to realize that the formation of sentences follows (grammatical) rules, and that the position of words within a sentence as well as their endings are affected by these rules. They begin to use plurals such as "shoes" and regular past tense verbs such as "jumped." From now on, speech development makes rapid progress, and language becomes an increasingly important tool in the daily interaction with family members. At age 4 years, the child should be able to understand most of the information imparted to him/her, and to follow even complex orders ("go to Daddy and tell him to come!"). Also, the child should be able to answer simple questions and recognize absurdities such as: "is that an elephant on the desk?" (Zollinger, 1996).

Before talking about speech development disorders, it is important to note that:

(1) there is great variation in the onset of expressive language.
(2) girls seem to develop the ability to communicate earlier than boys.
(3) language can develop smoothly and continuously, or in jumps and spurts.

Because the development of speech varies, it is inadequate to compare one child's language to the language of another. If a child's development of either receptive or expressive language is suspected to be delayed, or if the child shows, deficits in language performance, then he/she should be referred to a professional who will assess the problem on a theoretical background and base the diagnosis on population-based data about the process of language acquisition.

Definition and epidemiology

Speech development disorders (SDD) include several speech-related problems that manifest themselves as late onset, slow progression, or an erroneous course of language development. In the most extreme form, language may even fail to appear. The immediate consequences of SDD are impaired and ineffective oral communication, but in the long run SDD may also adversely affect an individual's scholastic performance, his/her development, and his/her social functioning.

An SDD is commonly considered a symptom (or complex of symptoms), resulting either from a neurological, audiological, genetic, psychiatric, etc. disease, or from adverse psychosocial conditions of the afflicted individual. In many cases, however, no underlying cause of the SDD can be identified.

Depending on how broadly or narrowly "SDD" is defined, its prevalence varies greatly: from 4% (Supacek and Simankova, 1982) over 10%–12% (Cantwell and Baker, 1987, 1997; Lahey, 1988) up to 25% (Heinemann and Höpfner, 1992, 2002), in recent publications from 4 to 8% (Grimm and Doil, 2000; Ruben, 2000) and for Specific Language Impairment (SLI) 6 to 8% (Tomblin et al., 1997, 1997a; Shafer et al., 2001; Grimm, 2003). Agreement exists that boys are more frequently affected than girls, the ratio being 2:1.

Classification

According to the traditional diagnostic approach, SDDs are categorized according to their (presumed) aetiology (organic versus functional). However, because aetiology is frequently uncertain, alternative classification schemes have been developed. To date, there exist several different classification schemes, none of which is generally accepted. Roughly, they can be divided into medical and linguistic schemes.

Medical classification schemes

ICD 10, Section F80–F89, provides diagnostic criteria for disorders of language development. In addition, the "phoniatric-pedaudiological" model, that is well

Table 3. Language development at different levels

Level	Examples
Phonological	Incorrect/inadequate use of sounds and syllables, problems with clarity of speech, pronunciation difficulties
Lexic & semantic	Limited availability of words and their meanings, poorly differentiated vocabulary
Syntactic	Irregular use of grammar, singular or short or incomplete sentences
Pragmatic	Poor communicative skills, only a few acts of speech available

established in the German-language countries, gives guidelines for SDD classification (Table 4). This model distinguishes between isolated SDDs (without concomitant disorder = Specific language impairment [SLI]) and complex SDDs

Table 4. Classification of childhood language disorders (mod. Kauschke and Siegmüller, 2002)

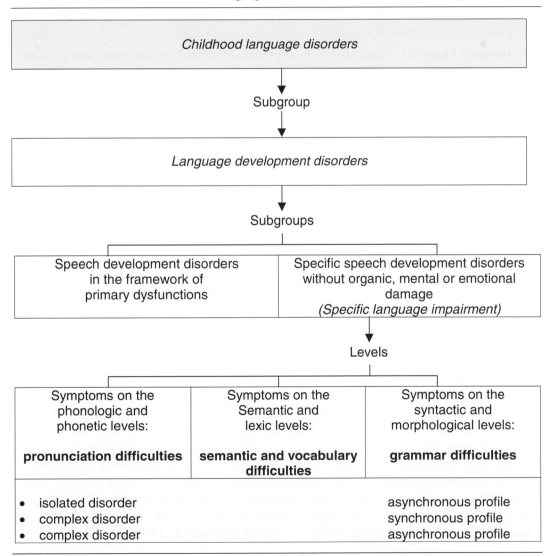

(in combination with organic or/and mental disorder). SDD can result from genetic disposition (hereditary), from organic defects (e.g. hearing impairment) or from adverse psychosocial factors (e.g. stimulus deprivation). Complex SDDs include diseases or disorders that affect organs crucial to normal speech and language development, e.g. epilepsy, cleft palate, or syndromes involving mental impairment.

Linguistic classification schemes

The linguistic approach characterizes SDDs according to the patholinguistic features of the impaired language. One of these models differentiates four different levels of speech performance and defines abnormal development according to how it affects each of the four levels. The levels are: (1) phonetic/ phonological, (2) morphological/syntactic, (3) lexic/semantic, and (4) pragmatic/ communicative (Table 3).

   After in-depth characterization of all deficits on each level, the language impairment is classified as:

- Isolated Disorder: one level (e.g. the syntactic one) is affected, while other levels develop normally.
- Comprehensive Disorder, synchronous type: all language levels are affected in a similar way.
- Comprehensive Disorder, asynchronous type: several levels are affected to varying degrees.

Another linguistic model distinguishes between impairment of articulation, impairment of semantics and vocabulary, and impairment of grammar.

Aetiology

Disorders or syndromes affecting the brain (cerebral paresis/MCD, dyspraxia, m. Down, cytomegaly, etc.) or the central nervous system (general growth retardation, motor diseases) frequently give rise to language acquisition problems. Sensory deprivation due to hearing impairment is another common aetiological factor. In addition, diseases or malformations of the speech organs (e.g. cleft palate, ankyloglossia) as well as psychiatric conditions (mental retardation, autism) must be considered as causes for a disturbed onset or course of language development.

   If no medical causes are found, social and psychological or psychiatric factors (Cantwell and Baker, 1997) must be taken into consideration. Bi- or multilingualism, with conflicting speech stimuli, can hinder smooth speech development. Poor or inadequate verbal stimulation due to insufficient social interaction affects the language of children who are frequently left alone (with TV or computer games as their main amusement) (Schröter, 2001) and of children whose parents are deaf-mute. Learning disabilities or emotional problems (e.g., separation anxiety, traumatic experiences) are still other reasons for a delayed onset or slow progression of speech (Zorowka, 1996).

In some children, none of the above aetiologies can be identified although it is known that other family members (e.g. parent, sibling, cousin) have or had similar problems with speech acquisition (Seemann, 1928; Tallal et al., 1989; Gopnik and Crago, 1991). This is a strong hint for a hereditary disposition, which may be involved in many SDD manifestations. In recent studies neuro-biological patterns are discussed as possibles causes: disorders or deviations of cell migration, nerve cell differentiation, of synaptogenesis and neural connection or metabolic disorders (Aram, 1991; Jernigan et al., 1991; Locke, 1994; Gauger et al., 1997; Gazzaniga, 2000; Shafer et al., 2001). In recent years research has identified several genes directly involved in language performance (Tomblin and Buckwalter, 1994; Gilger, 1995; Bishop et al., 1995; Bishop, 1997; Lai et al., 2000; Warbarton et al., 2000; Lai, 2001). However, a clear picture of the complex relationship between the genetic basis of speech (genotype) and its various phenotypical anomalies has not yet been drawn. To date, the "multi-factor/multi-effect" model is broadly accepted as a framework for understanding the genesis of language disorders (Kiese-Himmel, 1999). According to this model, a complex variety of biological factors (genetic disposition, neural functioning, . . .), psychological factors (cognitive abilities, personality features, . . .) and social factors (verbal stimulation, . . .) act together to promote the process of language acquisition. Each of them can be disturbed in different ways, and the effects of the disturbances can be manifold and difficult to predict.

It is an open question whether the specific language impairment (SLI) is a uniform developmental disorder or whether their subtypes reflect dysfunctions of certain language processing systems. Realisation of a genetic disposition aggravated by prenatal migration disorders is conceivable. To answer this question the expectations are now directed towards neurobiological and genetic markers.

Diagnosis

Due to the complex nature and diverse origins of SDDs, their diagnosis requires the cooperation of several professionals. Physicians, psychologists and speech pathologists need to work closely together, with the physician focusing on the possible medical cause of the language problem, the psychologist on the child's psychological and social conditions, and the speech pathologist on the features of the impaired language. A child with SDD should be referred to a specialist as early as possible: the earlier the problem is identified, the better the chance of repairing, correcting, or compensating a defect, and of conceptualising problem solutions in order to keep the consequences of the language disorder to a minimum (Kiese-Himmel, 1999; Ritterfeld and Niebuhr, 2002).

Anamnesis

Starting with pregnancy and birth, all precarious events in the life of the child should be determined: maternal diseases during pregnancy, maternal drug or alcohol abuse, problems during delivery (asphyxia) or afterwards (jaundice);

the child's diseases, ear problems, hospital stays, accidents, etc. Next, the development of his/her motor system, his/her previous language (including the preverbal phase), and his/her learning behavior must be discussed, because disturbances in these areas may indicate a more general problem. Then, the child's social interaction (siblings, family situation, contacts to playmates, . . .) should be analyzed, and signs of emotional distress (separation anxiety, problems falling asleep, fear of going to school, etc.) should be noted.

Clinical assessment

Clinical assessment includes three components: (1) The general assessment is performed by a pediatrician, who looks for general medical conditions that can contribute to SDDs (growth retardation, metabolic disorders, neurological diseases, syndromes, etc.). (2) The specific assessment is performed by a phoniatrician or pediatric otolaryngologist, whose examination directly addresses those organs and mechanisms involved in the production or processing of language. (3) Additional specific assessment by other medical specialists (e.g. ophthalmologists, oral surgeons, neurologists, psychiatrists, . . .) may be necessary if there are any hints that the SDD may be linked to a specific non-otolaryngological problem.

Most importantly, the hearing of the child must be assessed, and a history of recurrent ear infections or repeated middle ear problems must be given particular attention (Schönweiler et al., 1998). To exclude a hearing loss, subjective tests (behavioral observation audiometry, visual reinforcement audiometry, pure tone audiometry), as well as "objective" tests (oto-acoustic emissions [OAE], impedance audiometry, electric response audiometry [ABR]) can be administered. If the child's peripheral hearing is in order, yet a central auditory processing disorder is suspected, the child's auditory perception must be tested: speech understanding in noise, sound localization, phoneme discrimination, auditory memory span, or sound discrimination should be assessed to determine whether an auditory dysfunction underlies the language problem. Apart from a hearing loss, malformation of speech organs (macroglossia, ankyloglossia), adenoids, or nerve lesions frequently contribute to an SDD. Also, dysfunction of the oro-dento-pharyngeal unit (velopharyngeal insufficiency, or dental occlusion problems, . . .) should be considered if distorted speech production is the predominant feature.

Assessment of language development

To obtain a picture of the child's developmental status of language performance, two approaches can be used: (1) the "spontaneous talk" approach and (2) the "speech/language test" approach.

(1) The examiner may initiate talk or play with the child, and look at his/her verbal and behavioral responses. Receptive language can be checked by asking questions or commands, and observing whether or not the child responds appropriately. Expressive language skills can be examined by prompting the child to produce verbal utterances and by analyzing them according to vocabulary, grammar or articulation criteria. The advantage of this "spontaneous talk"

method is that the examiner is able to directly address the language deficits the child is supposed to exhibit. In a more elaborate way, the child's behavior can be recorded on video and audio tapes, and an in-depth analysis of his/her language skills can be performed.

(2) A more standardized approach to analyzing a child's language performance deficits is to subject him/her to speech tests. This is commonly done by language development professionals (developmental psychologists, speech therapists). A variety of tests for children from aged 2 or 3 years are available for assessing particular skills involved in the comprehension and production of language: sound (phoneme) production, sound (phoneme) discrimination, vocabulary, use of syntactic rules, verbal-auditory memory, comprehension of spatial or temporal concepts, understanding of complex sentences, etc.

Screening tests allows the identification of children at risk as early as aged 12 to 24 months (Grimm et al., 1996; Grimm and Doil, 2000) and standardized tests for german speaking children up to school age (SETK 2, SETK 3–5 [Grimm et al., 2001]).

The advantage of the "testing" approach to SDDs is that the child's skills can be quantified and compared to those of the age-matched population. This allows an objective and examiner-independent statement on the degree of language impairment (Schöler, 1999; Ritterfeld and Niebuhr, 2002).

Psychological assessment

Because of the close connection between language, intellectual skills and mental development, the psychological assessment of a child with SDD is indispensable. Deficits in or retardation of the mental, cognitive or emotional functions seriously interfere with language acquisition and need to be addressed by adequate therapeutic measures. Poor intelligence, learning disabilities, or mental impairment due to disorders or syndromes (m. Down, fragile X syndrome, cri-du-chat syndrome, Rett syndrome, etc.) regularly give rise to impaired language acquisition. Verbal and non-verbal intelligence tests and tests to assess specific cognitive abilities (concentration, awareness, memory, etc.) may be necessary to identify deficits in particular areas of cognitive functioning. Emotional problems presenting as sleep disturbances, unfounded anxieties, unwillingness to go to school, little social contact, or the like need to be addressed by a professional and must be tackled if measures to support language acquisition are to be successful. In addition, the family situation must be analyzed to find out if unfavourable interrelationships between family members are adversely affecting the child's socio-emotional development (e.g. parent questionnaires [Grimm and Doil, 2000]).

Treatment

As with diagnosis, the treatment of SDDs requires the collaboration of a multidisciplinary team of professionals: pediatricians, otolaryngologists, psychologists, speech therapists, teachers, psychiatrists, and – most importantly – parents. While each of these takes over a particular part of the treatment program, optimal coordination of their efforts and activities is mandatory. This requires good communication between professionals, on the one hand, and between professionals and parents, on the other hand. Also a well-elaborated therapeutic concept, which is known and supported by all involved persons, is helpful.

Treatment of SDD has three components: causal, habilitative and supportive. Causal treatment aims at repairing defects, correcting dysfunctions, or eliminating factors that – directly or indirectly – contribute in a causal way to the language problem. For instance, in the case of a hearing loss, hearing aids need to be fitted. In the case of emotional distress, the child must be helped to find emotional stability. In the case of concentration difficulties, the child needs awareness training. In some cases, surgery may be required (cleft palate, oromandibular malformation), while in others the treatment of the primary disease (e.g. a neurological or metabolic disorder) is paramount.

Habilitative treatment of SDDs, on the other hand, aims to directly improve the child's language skills. Appropriate measures include the extensive counselling of parents, who must be instructed to actively engage in their child's language development. Communication between them and the child must be enhanced, and they must be motivated to spend sufficient time verbally interacting with the child (e.g. telling stories, talking, playing together) or in performing specific exercises (reading, pronouncing, etc.) with him/her. Speech therapy provided by a professional is the most specific means of counteracting the child's language deficits. Professional speech therapy is indispensable in cases of severe speech development retardation, or in the presence of factors that make unaided speech acquisition impossible (e.g., oromandibular malformation).

In addition to the above treatments, supportive measures to boost language acquisition can be provided, if appropriate. For instance, training programs for speech-related skills (e.g. sound discrimination, memory, fine motor skills) may be implemented. Social contacts of the child to persons outside the family must be recognized as an important vehicle of language learning. Thus, attending playgroups or hobby clubs is recommended for children who would otherwise spend much time alone. Particular attention should be given to his/her situation at school. Teachers must be informed of any therapeutic measures and, if possible, should be involved in the treatment program.

In treating children with SDD, early initiation of the interventional measures is currently seen to be crucial. Not long ago, the "late bloomer" hypothesis was the dominant view among language experts. According to this hypothesis, a delay in early speech acquisition is no reason to worry, as 30% to 50% of affected children make up for it before age 3 to 4 years and subsequently exhibit normal language performance. "Wait and see" is the conclusion drawn from this view: treatment is necessary only if the language delay continues beyond age 4 years. The "late bloomer" hypothesis, however, is not undisputed (Ritterfeld, 2000; Kiese and Himmel, 1999a). While a certain percentage of developmentally delayed children indeed make up for their deficits without any intervention, a large percentage of them do not. At an early stage of development, however, it is impossible to predict whether or not a child is a "late bloomer". The "wait-and-see" strategy is thus disadvantageous for those children, whose deficits do not disappear on their own. As they do not benefit from early intervention, they are at risk to experience problems at school and show poor academic performance. Contrary to the "late bloomer" hypothesis, we suggest that SDDs be treated as soon as the first signs of problems in language acquisition manifest themselves (Kauschke and Konopatsch, 2001; Kauschke and Siegmüller, 2002).

Why is early intervention essential? There are several reasons.

Firstly, the acquisition of speech is a high-grade organized process, that occurs in an ontogenetically determined order of steps. Each step needs to be completed before the next one can be started. Defective or incomplete performance of one step poses problems for all subsequent steps. A problem occurring at an early level will thus affect a large number of developmental steps. In this regard, early intervention prevents the multiplication of a problem and minimizes its effect on the succeeding developmental levels (Bishop, 1997; Kuhl et al., 1992).

Secondly, speech acquisition follows an innate time schedule. Far from being a purely receptive process, which can take place at different ages, speech acquisition is complex interaction between genetically determined "sensitive phases" and environmental stimulation. Sensitive phases occur at specific ages and are committed to particular elements of speech: e.g. the recognition/production of sounds and phonemes, the sensitivity for prosodic features, the comprehension of syntactic structures, etc. (Zollinger, 1996). Each element of speech is best learned within its "sensitive phase". If developmental problems arise, early intervention can help ensure that sensitive phases are not missed or that the environmental stimuli are provided at a time that is not too distant from the sensitive phase.

Thirdly, language development is also essential to the development of a child's personality, to the development of his/her cognitive and social skills, and thus to the integrity of his/her future chances to cooperate and compete with others in an increasingly demanding world. Language is one of the most important tools of every individual and consequently should be given the greatest attention. Ignoring problems in its acquisition could give the child a life-long stigma and destroy many of his/her perspectives for a successful life. Although SDDs cannot be effectively treated, namely eliminated, in many children, their manifestations can nevertheless be mitigated and their consequences minimized. Early, appropriate and consequent treatment is the best way to present a speech development disorder from becoming a disability.

Conclusion

Impaired language development counts as a risk factor in the further cognitive and psychological development of the child, for acquiring the secondary verbal performances in reading and writing during its career in school. Therefore, early identification of disordered language development in the first years of life is of special importance.

References

Aram DM (1991) Comments on specific language impairment as a clinical category. Lang Speech Hear Serv Schools 22: 84–88

Bishop DVM (1997) Uncommon understanding, development and disorders of language comprehension in children. Psychology Press, Hove

Bishop DVM, North T, Donlan C (1995) Genetic basis of specific language impairment: evidence from a twin study. Dev Med Child Neurol 37: 56–71

Cantwell DP, Baker L (1987) Developmental speech and language disorders. Guilford Press, New York

Cantwell DP, Baker L (1997) Psychiatric disorders in children with speech and language retardation. Arch Gen Psychiatry 34: 583–591

Cantwell DP, Baker L, Mattison RE (1979) The prevalence of psychiatric disorder in children with speech and language disorder. J Am Acad Child Adolesc Psychiatry 18: 451–461

Gauger LM et al. (1997) Brain morphology in children with specific language impairment. J Speech Language Hearing Res 40: 1772–1784

Gazzaniga MS (2000) The new cognitive neurosciences. MIT Press, Massachusetts

Gilger JW (1995) Behavioral genetics: concepts for research and practice in language development and disorders. J Speech Hear Res 38: 1126–1142

Gopnik M, Crago MB (1991) Familial aggregation of a developmental language disorder. Cognition 39: 1–50

Grimm H (2003) Störungen der Sprachentwicklung, 2.Aufl. Hogrefe, Bern

Grimm H, Doil H (2000) ELFRA. Elternfragebogen für die Früherkennung von Risikokindern. Handanweisung. Hogrefe, Göttingen

Grimm H, Doil H, Müller C, Wilde S (1996) Elternfragebogen für die differentielle Erfassung früher sprachlicher Fähigkeiten. Sprache & Kognition 15: 32–45

Grimm H, Aktas M, Frevert S (2001) Sprachentwicklungstest für drei-fünfjährige Kinder (SETK 3–5). Hogrefe, Göttingen

Heinemann M, Höpfner C (1992) Screening-Verfahren zur Erfassung von Sprachentwicklungsstörungen (SEV) im Alter von 31/2 bis 4 Jahren bei der U8. Kinderarzt 23: 1635–1638

Heinemann M, Höpfner C (2002) Häufigkeit von Sprachentwicklungsverzögerungen bei dreieinhalb- bis vierjährigen Kindern. In: Gross M, Kruse E (Hrsg) Aktuelle phoniatrisch-pädaudiologische Aspekte 2002/2003, Bd 10. Median-Verlag, Heidelberg, S363–S366

Jernigan T, Hesselink JR, Sowell E, Tallal P (1991) Cerebral structure on magnetic resonance imaging in language- and learning-impaired children. Arch Neurol 48: 539–545

Kauschke C, Konopatsch S (2001) Einstieg in die Grammatik – Entwicklung über das Verblexikon. L.O.G.O.S. Interdisziplinär 9: 280–292

Kauschke C, Siegmüller J (2002) Patholinguistische Diagnostik bei Sprachentwicklungsstörungen. Urban & Fischer, München Jena

Kiese-Himmel C (1999) Ein Jahrhundert Forschung zur gestörten Sprachentwicklung. Sprache-Stimme-Gehör 23: 128–137

Kiese-Himmel C (1999a) Überlegungen zur psychologischen Frühdiagnstik von Sprachentwicklungsstörungen. Kindheit und Entwicklung 8: 92–99

Kuhl PK, Williams KA, Lacerda F, Stevens KN, Lindblom F (1992) Linguistic experience alters phonetic perception in infants by 6 months of age. Science 255: 606–608

Lahey M (1988) Language disorders and language development. Macmillan, New York

Lai CS (2001) A forkhead domain gene is mutated in a severe speech and language disorder. Nature 413: 519–523

Lai CS et al. (2000) The $SPCH_1$ region and human 7q31: genomic characterization of the critical interval and localization of translocations associated with speech and language disorder. Am J Hum Genet 67: 357–368

Locke JL (1994) Gradual emergence of developmental language disorder. J Speech Hear Res 37: 608–616

Ritterfeld U (2000) Zur Prävention bei Verdacht auf eine Spracherwerbsstörung: Argumente für eine gezielte Interaktionsschulung der Eltern. Frühförderung interdisziplinär 19: 80–87

Ritterfeld U, Niebuhr S (2002) Neue Wege in der Sprachentwicklungsdiagnostik. Kinder- und Jugendarzt 33: 321–329

Rosetti LM (2001) Communication intervention. Birth to three, 2nd edn. Singular Publishing Group/Thomson Learning, San Diego London

Ruben RJ (2000) Redefining the survival of the fittest: communication disorders in the 21st century. Laryngoscope 110: 241–245

Schöler H (1999) IDIS – Inventar diagnostischer Informationen bei Sprachentwicklungsauf-fälligkeiten. "Edition S" – Universitätsverlag Winter, Heidelberg

Schönweiler R, Ptok M, Radü HJ (1998) A cross-sectional study of speech- and language-abilities of children with normal hearing, mild fluctuating conductive hearing loss, or moderate to profound sensoneural hearing. Int J Pediatr Otorhinol Laryngol 44: 251–258

Schröter M (2001) Freizeitverhalten und familiäre Sozialisationsbedingungen sprachbehinderter und nicht sprachbehinderter Grundschulkinder im Vergleich. Sprachheilarbeit 46: 170–178

Seemann M (1928) Sprachstörungen bei Kindern. VEB Verlag Volk und Gesundheit, Berlin

Shafer VL et al. (2001) Neurophysiological indices of language impairment in children. Acta Otolaryngol 121: 297–300

Tallal P, Ross R, Curtiss S (1989) Familial aggregation in specific language impairment. J Speech Hear Disord 54: 167–173

Tomblin JB, Buckwalter P (1994) Studies of the genetics of specific language impairment. In: Watkins R, Rice M (eds) Specific language impairments in children. Brookes, Baltimore, pp 17–35

Tomblin JB, Records NL, Buckwalter P, Zhang X, Smith E, O'Brien M (1997) Prevalence of specific language impairment in kindergarten children. J Speech Lang Hear Res 40: 1245–1260

Tomblin JB, Smith E, Zhang X (1997) Epidemiology of specific language impairment: prenatal and perinatal risk factors. J Commun Disord 30: 325–344

Warbarton P et al. (2000) Support for linkage of autism and specific language impairment to 7q3 from two chromosome rearrangements involving band 7q31. Am J Med Genet 96: 228–234

Zoll B (1999) Genetik der Sprachentwicklungsstörungen. Stimme Sprache Gehör 23: 138–142

Zollinger B (1996) Die Entdeckung der Sprache, 2. Aufl. Haupt, Bern Stuttgart Wien

Zorowka P (1996) Sprachentwicklungsstörungen -eine neue Zivilisationskrankheit? Universitas 51/604: 940–954

Author's address: P. G. Zorowka, MD, Department for Hearing, Speech and Voice Disorders, Medical University Innsbruck, Anichstrasse 35, 6020 Innsbruck, Austria, e-mail: patrick.zorowka@uibk.ac.at

Disorders of motor development (clumsy child syndrome)

H. Sigmundsson

Research Group for Child Development, Department of Sociology
and Political Science, Norwegian University of Science and Technology,
Trondheim, Norway

Summary. This presentation will focus on motor competence, the clumsy child, perceptual deficits in clumsy children and possible neurological dysfunction in this group of children. Motor competence not only allows children to carry out everyday practical tasks, but it is also an important determinant of their level of self-esteem and of their popularity and status in their peer group. Research has shown that about 6–10% of children have motor competences well below the norm. It is unusual for motor problems to simply disappear over time. In the absence of intervention the syndrome is likely to manifest itself. In the clinical literature attempts have been made to establish causal links between surface manifestations of clumsiness and underlying perceptual deficits. In this respect the attention is primarily directed towards the concept of inter- and intra-modal matching, particularly with respect to vision and proprioception, an ability deemed to underlie many real-life motor skills. Neurobehavioural model of inter- and intra-modal matching and deficit model is presented. Findings from studies using this paradigm are discussed and it is argued that clumsiness must be seen as a neurological dysfunction (insufficiency).

Introduction

This overview article will focus mainly on the importance of motor competence for children, the clumsy child and perceptual deficits in clumsy children. Neurobehavioral model of inter- and intra-model matching and deficit model will be presented. Findings from studies using inter- and intra-modal matching paradigm and visual sensitivity tests will be presented and discussed in relation to the deficit model.

Motor competence

It is possible to argue that motor competence can be understood as the person's ability to carry out different motor skills. Research indicates that motor competence not only allows children to carry out everyday practical tasks (Henderson and Sugden, 1992), but it is also an important determinant of their level of self-esteem (Losse et al., 1991; Henderson, 1992) and of their popularity and status in their peer group (Leemrijse, 2000). By observing a child with dysfunctional movements who has problems making even the simplest movements, we become aware of the complexity of various processes an act of coordination involves. When a child starts school, it is expected to show proficiency in several skills that are necessary to function at home and school. In that age, the child is expected to be able to carry out manual dexterity tasks such as tying shoelaces, doing up buttons, using scissors, managing knife and fork, dressing, handwriting and drawing. Performance in gross motor tasks such as running, hopping and jumping is also important for the children to be able to do. Motor competence, in other words, will be of particular importance for a child who wants to meet the demands of the everyday life.

There is little research on motor competence of 'normal' children and adolescents. The reason for this is that available tests are sensitive to only one ends of the scale, in other words, they are designed for those who have low performance. Researchers main aim has been to create tests that will allow intercepting children with the lowest level of motor competence, to follow up their development and suggest treatment (see, for example, Henderson and Sugden, 1992).

While many studies have shown a significant correlation between motor problems and other problems in the social sphere, it has been difficult to establish causal relationships with any degree of confidence, as there appear to be several interactions which need to be taken into account. Research has shown that about 6–10% of children have motor competences well below the norm.

Clumsy children

Clumsiness is a concept that has been discussed in the literature for at least 75 years (e.g. Orton, 1937; Walton et al., 1962; Morris and Whiting, 1971; Gubbay, 1975; Gordon and McKinley, 1980; Henderson and Hall, 1982; Sigmundsson et al., 1997a; Sigmundsson and Hopkins, 2004).

As a behavioural phenomenon, however, the clumsiness syndrome must have been observed since time immemorial, much to the frustration of both parents and members of the medical profession confronted by children exhibiting the syndrome:

> This account would seem to describe my son who is $5\frac{1}{2}$ years old. His poor co-ordination has affected him socially for at least the last two years. A year ago, I took him for a check-up at the local cerebral palsy clinic which is all there is available in this area. The doctor didn't even examine him and only casually watched him walk in and then said he was perfectly normal in all respects. Granted he is within 'normal' limits! However, there has always been 'something slightly off'. He falls constantly without being aware of why – small muscle co-ordination is poor – it's difficult for him to hold a pencil (Morris and Whiting, 1971, p. 38–39)[1].

What then, it might be asked, is the extent reference of the term *motor impairment* when it has been used as a synonym for clumsiness (Orton, 1937); developmental dyspraxia (Dencla, 1984); developmental apraxia and agnosia

---

[1] Personal communication in a letter from an American parent whose child exhibited a 'clumsiness' syndrome

(Gubbay, 1975) and, most recently, developmental co-ordination disorder – DCD (APA, 1994)? Some of these categories have been further delineated. Apraxia, for example, has been classified as ideational when the defective performance of sequences of gestures is the observed deficit and as ideomotor when disturbance is confined to isolated gestures (Dewey, 1995). Whatever the label attached, however, there is agreement that the syndrome manifests itself '… as a level of competence in motor skills … significantly below the norm' (Henderson and Hall, 1982) – a description that is captured, albeit superficially, by the definition of *clumsiness* put forward by Morris and Whiting (1971) 'maladaptive motor behaviour in relation to expected or required movement performance'. Other authors who have tried to come to terms with the essential nature of this syndrome have found the need to be more circumspect and constrained in order to distinguish the phenomenon from more clearly diagnosable syndromes like, for example, cerebral palsy. Henderson and Hall (1982), qualify their definition of clumsiness by adding the rider '… but who show no evidence of disease of the nervous system' – a rather all-embracing and difficult to establish, exclusion criterion.

More recently, The American Psychiatric Association has coined the term 'Developmental Co-ordination Disorder (DCD)' to indicate a marked impairment in the development of motor co-ordination that is not explainable by mental retardation and is not due to a known physical disorder (APA, 1994). They apparently saw no reason to add a further qualification with respect to diseases (malfunctioning?) of the nervous system.

Basically, the implication in most of these definitions, as well as in the citation from the parent of such a child cited above, is that the clumsy child can be described as one who is clumsy in motor behaviour, but otherwise appears to be normal (Smyth, 1992). While there would seem to be reasonable agreement about the behavioural nature of the clumsiness syndrome there is little consensus with respect to causation. The aetiology has generally been couched in terms of nature versus nurture, most theoretical positions assigning at least some role to both but varying in the emphasis placed on either (Haywood, 1993; Berk, 1997; Sigmundsson and Whiting, 2002).

Where these issues have been pursued, the focus has been on pre-, peri- and post-natal factors (for a review, see Morris and Whiting, 1971). The possibility of peri-natal antecedents, in the earlier medical literature, led to the introduction of the terms 'minimal brain damage' (MBD) and 'minimal brain dysfunction'. Later, these terms were considered not only to be pejorative and, hence, politically unacceptable but also as not being very helpful and probably counterproductive with respect to designing and instigating intervention programmes. Dare and Gordon (1970, p. 178) insisted that '… there is no doubt that in many instances brain damage is present' and Gubbay (1975) and Hadders-Algra (2000) later argued that a continuum of neurological damage underlies the motor-impairment and that there is some overlap between cerebral palsy and clumsiness.

The drift away from neurological explanations post 1970's has been reflected in the nature and evolution of those tests devised to assess the degree of 'clumsiness' in children over wide age ranges. There has also been a noticeable

shift of attention away from tests designed with brain damage and/or dysfunction in mind (e.g. The Bender Gestalt test (Bender, 1938); Memory for Designs
test (Graham and Kendall, 1960)) towards more functionally oriented tests at
the level of surface behaviour. This is surprising given that some of the most
extensively used tests of clumsiness – like the ABC test of Henderson and
Sugden (1992) – stem from Stott's, 1966 test of motor impairment (Stott,
1966) which, in turn, is based on Gollnitz's (1960) revision of the Oseretsky
test (Oseretsky, 1923). Stott's main criterion for item selection was that motor
disability should be reasonably attributable to neural dysfunction, albeit on the
behavioural criterion of a failure to control or coordinate simple actions in the
absence of discernable physical disability (Morris and Whiting, 1971, p. 171).
One consequence of this development has been the restriction of much of the
earlier work on clumsiness (the work on *abilities* addressed below being an
exception) to descriptive studies at the level of observable behaviour, a trend
that might be seen to be unfortunate in the light of Stott's standpoint.

Prevalence and characteristics

The 6–10% estimate of the number of school-age children in Norway manifesting the clumsiness syndrome[2] (Søvik and Mæland, 1986; Mæland, 1992;
Sigmundsson et al., 1997a, 1999a) is very similar to the estimates made in other
countries (Brenner et al., 1967; Gubbay, 1975; Henderson and Hall, 1982). It is
unusual for motor problems to simply disappear over time. In the absence of
intervention the syndrome is likely to manifest itself. More recent research
points to some of the circularity in this causal network, children with motor
problems having been shown to be less physically active that their peers. In a
larger health perspective this in itself can have very serious consequences.

Children with low level of motor competence have low status among their
peers and low self-image (Losse et al., 1991; Henderson, 1992; Mæland, 1992;
Schoemaker and Kalverboer, 1994). Research shows connection between motor
problems and other problems, for example, problems with concentration, low
self-respect and emotional dysfunction (Henderson, 1992; Losse et al., 1991;
Schoemaker and Kalverboer, 1994).

A child with motor problems may end up in an evil circle that can even
lead to exclusion from games that, in turn, contributes to a negative self-image
(Bouffard et al., 1996). According to Harter (1987), as a result of repeated
unsuccessful attempts, children with motor problem have low level of physical
development. If these children do not participate in physical activity possibilities for development of new skills and participation in social environment with
other children will be limited. Less play, with or without other children, will
hinder successful development of motor competence due to limited practical
experience (Henderson, 1992). This indicates that motor competence of a

---

[2] Given that, at the surface level, clumsiness is characterised by deficiency in the performance of
fine and/or gross motor skills evidenced by, for example, a lack of manual dexterity in one or
more tasks such as tying shoelaces, doing up buttons, using scissors, managing a knife and fork,
dressing, handwriting and drawing, and/or deficiencies in skills of walking, running, hopping
etc., behavioural tests of the syndrome have focused on these classes of skill

particular child has implications for both social and emotional sides of everyday life, and not only in the sphere of the physical development and movement (Skinner and Piek, 2001).

Research has also shown that motor problems are connected with gender, and that boys often have a lower level of motor competence than girls. Gender differences vary from 2:1 to 10:1 (Gillberg et al., 1982). This means that the part of those who have motor problems varies from double as many boys as girls to ten times as many boys as girls.

Perceptual deficits in clumsy children

Over the last 30 years, psychologists have attempted to find explanations for inadequacies in motor performance by a search for deficits in the various cognitive processes involved in the planning and execution of movements (Henderson, 1992).

In the clinical literature, following Fleishman's (1966) approach, attempts have also been to establish causal links between surface manifestations of clumsy behaviour and, underlying perceptual abilities (Dare and Gordon, 1970; Laszlo and Bairstow, 1985).

Two particular perceptual modes, have attracted most attention, namely, the visual-perceptual and/or visual-motor deficits (Gubbay et al., 1965; Dare and Gordon, 1970; Henderson and Hall, 1982; Hulme et al., 1982a; Hulme et al., 1982b, 1984; Hulme and Lord, 1986; Powell and Bishop, 1992) and proprioceptive[3] deficits (Bairstow and Laszlo, 1981; Laszlo and Bairstow, 1985; Laszlo et al., 1988; Smyth, 1991, 1994). Exploring the perceptual deficiencies underlying movement coordination problems has been an encouraging line of inquiry, but limitations in the theoretical frameworks in which they have been formulated have mitigated against the usefulness and applicability of the findings. Much of the studies have been confined to the level of description with no consensus of opinion as to the underlying causal agencies (see for an overview Sigmundsson, 2003).

The idea that inter-modal (visual/proprioceptive) and intra-modal (proprioceptive/proprioceptive) matching might provide insight into the nature of the clumsiness syndrome was proposed in an investigation (unpublished) carried out by Jongmans (1989) and cited in Henderson (1993). Using a paradigm that Hofsten and Rösblad (1988) originally used with normal children, they investigated the performance of children exhibiting clumsy behaviour on a manual matching task to locate a target when the availability of vision and proprioception were systematically manipulated. Matching the located targets was always carried out without vision i.e. under proprioceptive control. Their results showed that wile the target remained visible the clumsy group performed as accurately as their control peers. When only proprioceptive information about target location was available, both groups were less accurate, but the decrease for the clumsy group was much more striking (Henderson, 1993).

---

[3] Proprioception: those receptor mechanisms, most noticeably in the joints, muscles and tendons, that signal information about the posture and movements of the body as a whole (Sherrington, 1906)

It was this kind of finding which led Sigmundsson et al. (1997a) to formulate a working neurobehavioral model of inter- and intra-modal matching into which the available data could be fitted and which might give rise to further predictions which would lend themselves to empirical testing.

Neurobehavioral model of inter- and intra-modal matching

Establishing the context for the model

The great commissure forms at once a bond of union and a band of separation (Wigan, 1844, in Bogen, 1990).

Bogen (1990) reiterates the words of Wigan in order to draw attention to the fact that although Sperry was awarded the Nobel Prize, as long ago as 1981, for his work with human split-brain subjects, the implications of this work have yet to be fully appreciated. In his words:

The principle of cerebral duality, first demonstrated in cats and monkeys and then confirmed in humans has so far had insufficient recognition' (Bogen, 1990, p. 215).

This by way of example is what Sperry said about human subjects in 1974:

Although some authorities have been reluctant to credit the disconnected minor hemisphere even with being conscious, it is our own interpretation – based on a large number and variety of nonverbal tests – that the other hemisphere is indeed a conscious system in its own right – perceiving, thinking, remembering, reasoning, willing, and emoting – all at a characteristically human level, and that both the left and right hemisphere may be conscious simultaneously in different, even mutually conflicting, mental experiences that run along in parallel (p. 11).

With respect to somatosensory information processing (touch, proprioception) it soon became clear that if a commisurotomised human was allowed to blindly feel a stimulus, then only the hemisphere contralateral to that hand was aware of the identity of the stimulus (see the review by Bogen, 1993). This kind of exercise illustrated that the pathways for the transmission of proprioceptive and haptic information are almost completely crossed (Galin et al., 1977, 1979; Geffen et al., 1985; Mima et al., 1999) the corpus callosum serving a mediating role in the interhemispheric transfer of information (Quinn and Geffen, 1986; Preilowski, 1972, 1990; Jeeves, 1990; Zaidel, 1998).

Inter-modal matching

Sandström (1953) and Sandström and Lundberg (1956), using groups of normal adults, and later Hofsten and Rösblad (1988) using groups of normal children in their experimental work, introduced an inter-modal condition (vision-proprioception) which for success demands congruency between the visual space and the proprioceptive space of the matching hand (see for review Hofsten and Rösblad, 1988). The hypothetical information-processing route when subjects are required to match information from visual space with the proprioceptive space of the left hand would, on the basis of current knowledge, appear to be as illustrated schematically in Fig. 1. For the right hand the projections would need to be mirror-imaged.

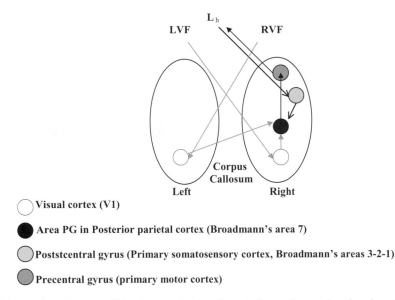

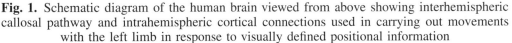

Fig. 1. Schematic diagram of the human brain viewed from above showing interhemispheric callosal pathway and intrahemispheric cortical connections used in carrying out movements with the left limb in response to visually defined positional information

From the right visual field (RVF) to the visual cortical projection area V1 in the left hemisphere and the left visual field (LVF) to a similar projection area (V1) in the right hemisphere, thereafter to area PG in the posterior parietal cortex (PPC) (Broadmann's area 7) – a polysensory, 'intermodal mixing area' considered to have a role in controlling spatially guided behaviour (Mountcastle et al., 1975; Robinson et al., 1978; Mishkin et al., 1983; Kolb and Whishaw, 1996). From area PG information projects onto the precentral gyrus (primary motor cortex) in the same hemisphere as that this controls the left hand (output). Feedback from the left hand, in turn, projects to the right postcentral gyrus (primary somatosensory cortex; Broadmann's areas 3–2–1), to area PG and is important for matching i.e. congruency between the visual space reference (system goal) and proprioceptive space of the matching hand (system output).

Intra-modal matching

If both hands are involved in an act, it is important that the information space defined by the one limb is in correspondence with the information space defined by the other (intra-modal matching). An example was provided by Laszlo and Bairstow (1980), using groups of both normal children and adults and, later, by Hofsten and Rösblad (1988) using groups of normal children in their study of proprioceptive-proprioceptive matching. The hypothetical route for such matching, based on current knowledge, would be seen to be that presented schematically in Fig. 2.

Information picked up via the right hand projects onto the postcentral gyrus (primary somatosensory cortex) in the left parietal lobe and is transmitted to the left posterior parietal cortex (PPC, Broadmann's areas 5 and 7) (Kolb and Whishaw, 1996) via the corpus callosum, to the posterior parietal cortex of the

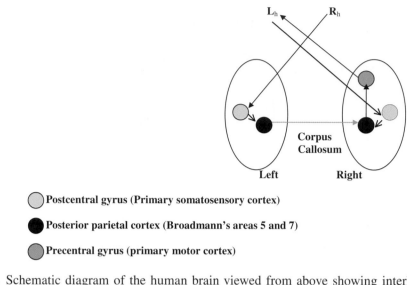

○ Postcentral gyrus (Primary somatosensory cortex)

● Posterior parietal cortex (Broadmann's areas 5 and 7)

● Precentral gyrus (primary motor cortex)

Fig. 2. Schematic diagram of the human brain viewed from above showing interhemispheric callosal pathway and intrahemispheric cortical connections used in carrying out movements with the left limb in response to proprioceptively defined positional information from right hand

opposite hemisphere; it traverses a pathway from there to the precentral gyrus (primary motor cortex) in the right hemisphere which controls the left hand (Geffen et al., 1985; Quinn and Geffen, 1986). The left hand is, in this case, used as a haptic[4] perceptual system (Gibson, 1966) – feedback from the hand projecting onto area PPC via the right postcentral gyrus providing the other input necessary for determining the congruency between the proprioceptive space of the right and the left hand in this comparator area.

For the right hand matching the projections would need to be mirror-imaged. Intra-modal matching might also be mediated 'intrahemispherically'. This, however, would require ipsilateral matching. As this cannot be done using the two hands one solution, introduced by Sigmundsson et al. (1999a) was to use the foot and hand of the same side. This also provided the possibility to locate the target in combination, felt and seen i.e. in case of left hand matching, the model would need to be a combination of Figs. 1 and 2.

Neurobehavioural models of the kind put forward lend themselves to questions about the effects that might be expected when communication between particular projection areas is impaired because of brain dysfunction or retardation in the establishment of the interconnections. Such impairment can be attributed to a 'delay' and/or 'deviancy' (neurological lesion/disconnection). Perturbations and predictions in this respect have been evident in the literature for almost a hundred years (see for review Bogen, 1993).

---

[4] 'This apparatus consists of a complex of subsystems. It has no 'sense organs' in the conventional meaning of the term, but the receptors in tissue are nearly everywhere and the receptors in the joints co-operate with them. Hence the hands and other body members are, in effect, active organs of perception . . . Touch and vision in combination often yield a redundant, double guaranteed input of information' (Gibson, 1966)

Deficit model

Delay versus deviancy

A recurring theme within the field of clumsiness has been the notion that discrepancies between the motor behaviour of clumsy and normal children can be seen as either manifesting delayed development or deviancy.

The apparently simple phrase 'motor delay' implies something quite different from the term 'developmental agnosia and apraxia' (Gubbay, 1975). Whereas the first seems to imply a rather benign condition which will disappear over time the second implies a condition which mirrors one that occurs in adults with known and irreversible brain damage (Losse et al., 1991; Barnett and Henderson, 1992). I will argue here that in the light of new theories within development (Gottlieb, 1998) and learning (Edelman, 1987, 1992) that the term 'motor delay' must be qualified and clumsiness must be seen as neurological dysfunction (Sigmundsson et al., 1997a, b, 1999a, b; Sigmundsson and Whiting, 2002; Sigmundsson, 2003).

Individual development

Theories within developmental psychology have normally been based upon theories within embryology (Connolly, 1970, 1986). The tendency have been that theories within developmental psychology have develop as the consequence of new knowledge and understanding within embryology and in less grade as a consequence of research within psychology. Maturation theories (Shirley, 1931; McGraw, 1935; Gesell, 1954) did dominate the field of developmental psychology until 1970, by that time it was challenged by researchers within the field (Connolly, 1970, 1986). In this period the current view within embryology did change, and the milieu did get a larger role in individual development. Gilbert Gottlieb comes with his probabilistic epigenesis theory around 1970 (Gottlieb, 1970, 1976). The probabilistic epigenesis theory focuses on the bidirectional nature of genetic, neural, behavioural and environmental influences on individual development.

Learning

The role of practice (learning) for individual development has received increased attention and, with it the role of nurture and environmental conditioning (Gottlieb, 1998; Edelman, 1987, 1992). The concept of development has become closely linked to the concept of learning (practice or experience leading to changes in the ability to perform tasks). This leads us to question the relative roles of nature and nurture in acquiring different skills. Edelman's theory (Edelman, 1987, 1992) on 'neural Darwinism' argues that learning can be explained as a selection within the neural system. The theory emphasis that stimuli and training increases connections within specific areas of the brain. Training strengthens the neural network which is used. Rostoft and Sigmundsson (2004) pointed out that it is possible to argue that Edelman's theory support the perspectives on 'task specificity' of learning.

Neurological dysfunction (insufficiency)

When taken these theories as an approach for understanding development and developmental disorder, clumsiness must be seen as a neurological dysfunction (insufficiency). This is earlier supported by a number of researchers that have pointed out that their findings with clumsy children could be behavioural manifestation of putative neurological disorders. Dare and Gordon (1970) interpret clumsiness as a part of the continuum of cerebral palsy. Gubbay (1975) also pointed out that clumsy children often have minor or uncertain neurological abnormalities and Dunn (1986) considered their impaired motor behaviour to be an aspect of the minimal brain damage (MBD) syndrome.

At the beginning of the century, Liepmann, ventured a hypothesis linking neurological disconnection to apraxia[5] (in Heilman and Rothi, 1993 and Bogen, 1993). According to this concept apraxia resulted from a disconnection of motor areas from sensory areas. The problem with this concept, even if confirmed, is that deficits resulting from a putative disconnection of areas are difficult to distinguish from similar deficits resulting from damage within one or other of the areas involved. Kolb and Whishaw (1996) pointed out in this respect that: 'As a result strict localisation of function becomes unworkable' (p. 12). It is not surprising, therefore, that Liepmann's hypothesis has more recently, been related both to intrahemispheric lesion/disconnection (Geschwind, 1975; Heilman and Rothi, 1993; Faglioni and Basso, 1985) and interhemispheric disconnection (Bogen, 1993).

It was this kind of distinction that prompted Sigmundsson and co-workers, beginning in 1997, to instigate a series of studies on clumsy children in which the methodology of inter-modal and intra-modal matching was used guided by the neurobehavioral models constructed for the purpose and illustrated in Figs. 1 and 2. The idea was to explore putative neurological explanations of clumsiness far more intensively.

Putative neurological dysfunction (insufficiency)

In the literature, there is universal agreement that children who are clumsy do not constitute a homogeneous group (Henderson and Sugden, 1992; Sigmundsson et al., 1997a). It would, therefore, seem much more meaningful and productive to focus on more clearly defined subgroups of children exhibiting clumsy behaviour and, at the same time, to go beyond the level of description to more explanatory frameworks. With this in mind Sigmundsson and his co-workers in a series of related studies turned their attention to a specific subcategory of clumsy children attending normal schools, namely, those exhibiting hand–eye coordination problems (HECP).

Test procedures developed in our laboratory for this purpose, in contrast to those that focus only on surface behaviour, have been directed towards this sensory integration abilities deemed to underlie the way in which these children carry out range of everyday motor tasks (Laszlo and Bairstow, 1985; Hofsten and Rösblad, 1988; Rösblad and Hofsten, 1992; Lee et al., 1990, 1997). In this

---

[5] Apraxia: inability to organise movements purposefully (Kalat, 1995)

way, parallels have been drawn between behavioural manifestations of 'clumsiness' and possible underlying neurological information processing disorder, which, in turn, has implications for the concept of hemispheric competence. This research has been made possible by the elaboration of an earlier developed testing instrument for sensory integration (Sandström, 1953; Sandström and Lundberg, 1956; Hofsten and Rösblad, 1988).

Sensory integration tests

1) Manual matching task: 'Inter- and intra-modal matching'

Basically, the testing procedures require the sensory matching of targets located visually (seen target), with the hand (felt target) or in combination (felt and seen). Matching of the position of located targets is normally carried out without vision – an exception being the Sigmundsson (1999) study.

Studies carried out using these testing procedures (Sigmundsson et al., 1997a, b; Sigmundsson, 1999) produced evidence of significant differences in inter- and intra-modal matching between right-handed HECP and normal children (age ranges 5–8 years) when combined scores for both hands were analysed. If Hofsten and Rösblad's (1988) and Lee et al. (1990, 1997) views are accepted, i.e. that competence in inter- and intra-modal matching are crucial to the acquisition and maintenance of motor skills, the deficiencies exhibited by the HECP groups, might be seen as a causal factor in their motor problems. Care, however, must be taken with such an interpretation because, as Hulme et al. (1982a) argue, it is difficult to pin-point whether the perceptual problems being demonstrated are the cause of the motor problems or if motor problems are the cause of the perceptual problems. This 'chicken-egg' problem remains a source of contention.

Analysis of the scores achieved with the right and left hand separately (see Table 1), however, demonstrated that the differences between the HECP and the control children could, in the main, be attributed to lowered performances when the left hand (non-preferred hand) was used for matching the located target position in the intra-modal (P) condition and in condition VP (felt and seen target). Within groups analyses produced evidence of significant asymmetrical differences in P and VP conditions in the HECP group only – matching with the right hand producing superior performance. In the inter-modal (V) condition the HECP children were significantly worse with both hands compared to their control groups (Sigmundsson et al., 1997a, b). It is important to note the absence of asymmetrical findings in this condition.

One of the limitations of the 'manual matching task', is that ipsilateral matching without vision is not possible making it difficult to pin-point more precisely the nature of the problems in the HECP group in condition P and VP and to be able to speculate about the cortical projection areas which may mediate in the transfer of information. Is it a left hemisphere input problem, an asymmetrical inter-hemispheric transfer problem or a deficit in processing information within the right hemisphere? This question led to the development of a new version of the task using toe-hand rather than hand-hand matching.

Table 1. Overview of studies on inter- and intra-modal matching by 7- and 8-year old children diagnosed as having hand–eye co-ordination problems (HECP) and by a control group of children without such problems

Study	Input	Output	P*	Possible explanations of the differences
Sigmundsson et al. (1997a, b)	vision (condition V) vision (condition V)	right hand left hand	s (mean AE) s (mean AE)	visual-perceptual and/or visual-motor deficits
Sigmundsson et al. (1997a, b)	vision/right hand (condition VP)	left hand	s (mean AE)	visual-perceptual and/or visual-motor deficits, problem which modality to rely on
Sigmundsson et al. (1997a, b)	vision/left hand (condition VP)	right hand	ns	
Sigmundsson et al. (1997a, b)	right hand (condition P)	left hand	s (mean AE)	right hemisphere insufficiency with or without dysfunctional corpus callosum
Sigmundsson et al. (1997a, b)	left hand (P)	right hand	ns	

* Significant (s) differences between the HECP and the control group of children on the mean absolute error (AE) score

2) HEMI-task: 'foot–hand' matching

This task, in principle, provides the possibility to distinguish between intra- and inter-hemispheric competences in intra-modal (proprioceptive) 'on-line' target location-matching. Using the foot rather than the hand to locate targets allows the possibility to examine performance when the information processing involved is within hemispheres as well as between hemispheres (a possibility which is not afforded when the hand is used for location and the other hand for matching) (Sigmundsson et al., 1999a). Such a procedure, it was thought, might provide a window into information-processing in the brain. The findings from a study (Sigmundsson et al., 1999a) carried out on a different group of seven year-old HECP children (right hand preferent) showed that they did manifest inferior performance to the control children in 3 of the 4 conditions where the right hemisphere was involved and/or information had to be transported across the corpus callosum.

Placed in the context of the neurobehavioral models presented, it is suggested that the findings from the manual matching task; condition P and VP; and from the foot–hand task could be accounted for by right hemispheric insufficiency (Geschwind, 1975; Faglioni and Basso, 1985; Heilman and Rothi, 1993) with or without a dysfunctional corpus callosum which, in turn, might be attributable to slow maturation (Yakolev and Lecours, 1967; Trevarthen, 1974; Galin et al., 1977; O'Leary, 1980; Quinn and Geffen, 1986) or an interruption of transcallosal interhemispheric communication – the so-called 'callosal concept' of Bogen (1993).

Visual sensitivity tests

The findings from the studies using inter- and intra-modal matching paradigm clearly indicate the problem HECP children have compared with their controls in the inter-modal matching condition, namely when the targets are located under visual control (see Table 1). In a follow-up study, Sigmundsson et al. (2003) compared visual processing by 10-year-old children diagnosed as having a clumsiness syndrome with controls on three different psychophysical tasks. These tasks involved global motion processing using a dynamic random dot kinematogram, static global pattern processing where the position of the target was randomised, and static global pattern processing in which the target position was fixed. The clumsy children were significantly less sensitive than the control group on all three tasks of visual sensitivity. Thus, clumsy children may have impaired visual sensitivity in both the dorsal and ventral streams.

It may be argued that inter- and intra-modal matching problems possible indicate a dorsal stream dysfunction. Sigmundsson and Hopkins (2004) followed up the possible ventral stream dysfunction and found that HECP children have a problem in visual recognition or more specifically the ability to identify a common object from an incomplete visual presentation as discerned by a test of visual closure. This finding also raises the possibility that the visual processing problems of clumsy children contribute to, or even strongly determine, not only their movement problems but also their learning difficulties as pointed out, earlier, by a number of researchers (Gubbay, 1975; Drillien and Drummond, 1983).

These findings from the sensory integration tests and the visual sensitivity tests might be speculated, could be a possible factor contributing to the problems that motor-impaired children are reported to encounter in more complex everyday fine-motor skills like needlework, dressing, doing up buttons and shoelaces etc. (for a review see Smyth, 1992) and in 'almost' every task when temporal constraints are imposed.

Conclusion

Motor competence not only allows children to carry out everyday practical tasks, but it is also an important determinant of their level of self-esteem and of their popularity and status in their peer group. Research has indicated that 6–10% of children have motor competences well below the norm. It is unusual for motor problems to simply disappear over time. In the absence of intervention the syndrome is likely to manifest itself.

Previous research involving clumsy children has been characterised by a focus on test outcomes (i.e. a product based approach), which simply describes the problems, but cannot explain them. To achieve the latter requires a process-orientated approach, which attempts by appropriate experimentation to tease out the ways in which these children organise their actions in time and space. This approach has been the departure point for recent research in our group.

Findings from our studies using the manual matching task; condition P and VP; and from the foot–hand task indicates that there is mainly problem when the left hand (nonpreferred hand) was used to match the position of the located target. Putative neurological disorder related to the development of the hemisphere controlling the left hand with/or without a dysfunctional corpus callosum are invoked to account for the poor performance with the left hand of the HECP children.

The inter-modal matching problem i.e. the problem in the integration between vision and proprioception may be related both to visual deficit and to proprioceptive problem. Clumsy children may have impaired visual sensitivity in both the dorsal and ventral streams in addition to their obvious problem with motor control. It is suggested that this findings are behavioural manifestations of a putative neurological dysfunction (insufficiency) (Sigmundsson et al., 1997a, b, 1999a, b; Sigmundsson, 1999, 2003; Sigmundsson and Whiting, 2002). This view is earlier supported by a number of researchers (Dare and Gordon, 1970; Gubbay, 1975; Dunn, 1986; Hadders-Algra, 2000).

References

American Psychiatric Association (1994) Diagnostic and statistical manual of mental disorders, 4th ed. American Psychiatric Association, Washington DC

Bairstow PJ, Laszlo JI (1981) Kinaesthetic sensitivity to passive movements in children and adults, and its relationship to motor development and motor control. Dev Med Child Neurol 23: 606–616

Barnett A, Henderson SE (1992) Some observations on the figure drawings of clumsy children. Br J Educ Psychol 62: 341–355

Bender AL (1938) A visual-motor Gestalt test. Res Monogr 3. NY Am Orthopsychiatr Assoc

Berk L (1997) Child development. Allyn and Bacon, MA

Bogen JE (1990) Parital hemispheric independence with the neocommissures intact. In: Trevarthen C (ed) Brain circuits and functions of the mind. Cambridge University Press, New York, pp 215–230

Bogen JE (1993) The Callsoal syndromes. In: Heilman KM, Valenstein R (eds) Clinical neuropsychology, 3rd ed. Oxford University Press, New York, pp 337–407

Bouffard M, Watkinson EJ, Thompson LP, Dunn JLC, Romanow SKE (1996) A test of the activity deficit hypothesis with children with movement difficulties. Adapt Phys Act Quart 13: 61–73

Brenner MW, Gillman S, Zangwill OL, Farrell M (1967) Visuo-motor disability in school-children. Br Med J 4: 259–262

Connolly KJ (1970) Skill development: problems and plans. In: Connolly KJ (ed) Mechanisms of motor skill development. Academic Press, London

Connolly KJ (1986) A perspective on motor development. In: Wade MG, Whiting HTA (eds) Motor development in children: aspects of coordination and control. Martinus Nijhoff, Dordrecht

Dare MT, Gordon N (1970) Clumsy children: a disorder of perception and motor organisation. Dev Med Child Neurol 12: 178–185

Dewey D (1995) What is developmental dyspraxia? Brain Cogn 29: 254–274

Drillien C, Drummond M (1983) Developmental screening and the child with special needs: a population study of 5000 children, Heinemann, London (Clin Dev Med 86)

Dunn HG (1986) Sequelae of low birthweight: the Vancouver study. Mac Keith Press with Blackwell Scientific; Lippincott, Philadelphia (Clin Dev Med 95/96)

Edelman GM (1987) Neural Darwinism. Basic Books, New York

Edelman GM (1992) Bright air, brilliant fire: on the matter of the mind. Basic Books, New York

Faglioni P, Basso A (1985) Historical perspectives on neuroanatomical correlates of limb apraxia. In: Roy EA (ed) Neuropsychological studies of apraxia and related disorders. Elsevier Science Publishers B.V., Amsterdam, pp 3–44

Fleishman EA (1966) Human abilities and the acquisition of skill. In: Bilodeau EA (ed) Acquisition of skill. Academic Press, New York, pp 147–167

Galin D, Diamond R, Herron J (1977) Development of crossed and uncrossed tactile localisation on the fingers. Brain Lang 4: 588–590

Galin D, Johnstone J, Nakel L, Herron J (1979) Development of the capacity for tactile information transfer between hemispheres in normal children. Science 204: 1330–1332

Geffen G, Nilsson J, Quinn K (1985) The effect of lesions of the corpus callosum on finger localisation. Neuropsychologia 4: 497–514

Geschwind N (1975) The apraxias: neural mechanisms of disorders of learned movement. Am Sci 63: 188–195

Gessel A (1954) The ontogenesis of infant behaviour. In: Carmichael L (ed) Manual of child psychology, 2nd ed. Wiley, New York

Gibson JJ (1966) The senses considered as perceptual systems. Houghton Mifflin, Boston

Gillberg C, Rassmussen P, Carlström G, Svenson B, Waldenström E (1982) Perceptual, motor and attentional deficits in six-year-old children. Epidemiological aspects. J Child Psychol Psychiatry 23: 131–144

Gollnitz G (1960) A revision of the Oseretsky Test of Motor Ability (unpublished)

Gordon N, McKinley I (1980) Helping clumsy children. Churchill Livingstone, Edinburgh

Gottlieb G (1970) Conceptions of prenatal development. In: Aronson LR, Tobach E, Lehrman DS, Rosenblatt JS (eds) Development and evaluation of behaviour: essays in memory of T. C. Schneirla. WH Freeman, San Francisco, pp 111–137

Gottlieb G (1976) Conceptions of prenatal development: behaviour embroyology. Psychol Rev 83: 215–234

Gottlieb G (1998) Normal occurring environmental and behaviuour influences on gene activity: from central dogma to propabilistic epigenesis. Psychol Rev 105: 792–802

Graham FK, Kendell BS (1960) Memory for designs test. Revised general manual. Percept Mot Skills 11: 147–188

Gubbay SS (1975) The clumsy child: a study of developmental and agnosic ataxia. Saunders, London

Gubbay SS, Ellis T, Walton JN, Court SDM (1965) Clumsy children: a study of apraxia and agnosic deficits in 21 children. Brain 88: 295–312

Hadders-Algra M (2000) The clumsy child – at the border of cerebral palsy? In: Velcikovic Peret M, Neville B (eds) Cerebral palsy. Elsevier Science, Amsterdam

Harter S (1987) The determinants and mediational role of global self-worth. I. Children. In: Eisenberg N (ed) Contemporary topics in developmental psychology. Wiley, New York, pp 219–242

Haywood KM (1993) Life span motor development. Human Kinetics Publishers, Champaign

Heilman KM, Rothi LJG (1993) Apraxia. In: Heilman KM, Valenstein R (eds) Clinical neuropsychology, 3rd ed. Oxford University Press, New York, pp 141–163

Henderson SE (1992) Clumsiness or developmental co-ordination disorder: a neglected handicap. Curr Paediatr 2: 158–162

Henderson SE (1993) Motor development and minor handicap. In: Kalverboer AF, Hopkins B, Geuze RH (eds) Motor development in early and later childhood. Longitudinal approaches. European Network on Longitudinal Studies on Individual Development (ENLS). Cambridge University Press, Cambridge

Henderson SE, Hall D (1982) Concomitants of clumsiness in young schoolchildren. Dev Med Child Neurol 24: 448–460

Henderson SE, Sugden D (1992) The movement assessment battery for children. The Psychological Corporation, Kent

Hofsten C von, Rösblad B (1988) The integration of sensory information in the development of precise manual pointing. Neuropsychologia 26: 805–821

Hulme C, Lord R (1986) Review clumsy children – a review of recent research. Child Care Health Dev 12: 257–269

Hulme C, Biggerstaff A, Moran G, McKinley I (1982a) Visual, kinaesthetic and cross-modal judgements of length by normal and clumsy children. Dev Med Child Neurol 24: 461–471

Hulme C, Smart A, Moran G (1982b) Visual perceptual deficits in clumsy children. Neuropsychologia 20: 475–481

Hulme C, Smart A, Moran G, McKinley I (1984) Visual, kinaesthetic and cross-modal judgements of length by clumsy children: a comparison with young normal children. Child Care Health Dev 10: 117–125

Jeeves MA (1990) Agenesis of the corpus callosum. In: Nebes RD, Corkin S (eds) Handbook of neuropsychology. Elsevier Science Publishers B.V., Amsterdam, pp 99–114

Jongmans M (1989) The relationship between perception and action in manual control of children with specific movement difficulties. Faculty of Human Movement Sciences. Free University, Amsterdam (unpublished)

Kalat JW (1995) Biological psychology. Brooks/Cole Publishing Company, USA

Kolb B, Whishaw IQ (1996) Fundamentals of human neuropsychology. W. H. Freeman and Company, New York

Laszlo JI, Bairstow PJ (1980) The measurement of kinaesthetic sensitivity in children and adults. Dev Med Child Neurol 22: 454–464

Laszlo JI, Bairstow PJ (1985) Perceptual motor behaviour: developmental assessment and therapy. Holt, Rinehart and Winston, London

Laszlo JI, Bairstow PJ, Bartrip J, Rolfe UT (1988) Clumsiness or perceptuo-motor dysfunction. In: Colley AM, Beech JR (eds) Cognition and action in skilled behaviour. Elsevier Science Publishers B.V., Amsterdam

Lee DN, Daniel BM, Turnball J, Cook ML (1990) Basic perceptuo-motor dysfunctions in cerebral palsy. In: Jennerod M (ed) Attention and performance. XIII. Motor representation and control. Erlbaum Associates, Hillsdale, pp 593–603

Lee DN, Hofsten C von, Cotton E (1997) Perception in action approach to cerebral palsy. In: Connolly KJ, Forssberg H (eds) Neurophysiology and neuropsychology of motor development. Mac Keith Press, London

Leemrijse C (2000) Developmental coordination disorder: evaluation and treatment. Free University, Amsterdam

Losse A, Henderson SE, Elliman D, Hall D, Knight E, Jongmans M (1991) Clumsiness in children. Do they grow out of it? A 10-year follow-up study. Dev Med Child Neurol 33: 55–68

Mæland AF (1992) Identification of children with motor coordination problems. Adapt Phys Act Quart 9: 330–342

McGraw MB (1945) The neuromuscular maturation of the human infant. Columbia University Press, New York

Mima T, Sadato N, Yazawa S, Hanakawa T, Fukuyama H, Yonekura Y, Shibasaki H (1999) Brain structures related to active and passive finger movements in man. Brain 122: 1989–1997

Mishkin M, Ungerleider LG, Macho KA (1983) Object vision and spatial vision: two cortical pathways. Trends Neurosci 6: 414–417

Morris PR, Whiting HTA (1971) Motor impairment and compensatory education. G Bell and Sons, Philadelphia

Mountcastle VB, Lynch JC, Georgopoulos A, Sakata H, Acuna CJ (1975) Posterior parietal association cortex of the monkey: command functions for operations within extrapersonal space. J Neurophysiol 38: 871–908

O'Leary DS (1980) A developmental study of interhemispheric transfer in children aged five to ten. Child Dev 51: 743–750

Orton ST (1937) Reading, writing and speech problems in children. Norton, New York

Oseretsky NI (1923) A metric scale for studying the motor capacity of children (in Russian)

Powell RP, Bishop DVM (1992) Clumsiness and perceptual problems in children with specific language impairment. Dev Med Child Neurol 34: 755–765

Preilowski B (1972) Possible contribution of the anterior forebrain commissures to bilateral co-ordination. Neuropsychologia 10: 267–277

Preilowski B (1990) Intermanual transfer, interhemispheric interaction, and handedness in man and monkeys. In: Trevarthen C (ed) Brain circuits and functions of the mind. Cambridge University Press, New York, pp 160–180

Quinn K, Geffen G (1986) The development of tactile transfer of information. Neuropsychologia 24: 793–804

Robinson DL, Goldberg ME, Stanton GB (1978) Parietal association cortex in the primate: sensory mehanisms and behavioural modulations. J Neurophysiol 41: 910–932

Rostoft MS, Sigmundsson H (2004) Developmental co-ordination disorder: different perspectives on the understanding of motor control and co-ordination. Adv Physiother 6: 11–19

Rösblad B, Hofsten C von (1992) Perceptual control of manual pointing in children with motor impairments. Physiother Theory Pract 8: 223–233

Sandström CI (1953) Sex differences in localisation and orientation. Acta Psychol 9: 82–96

Sandström CI, Lundberg I (1956) A genetic approach to sex differences in localisation. Acta Psychol 12: 247–253

Schoemaker MM, Kalverboer AF (1994) Social and affective problems of children who are clumsy: how early do they begin? Adap Phys Act Quart 11: 130–140

Sherrington CS (1906) The integrative action of the nervous system. Yale University Press, New Haven

Shirley MM (1931) The first two years: a study of twenty-five babies, vol 1. Postual and locomotor development. University of Minnesota Press, Minneapolis

Sigmundsson H (1999) Inter-modal matching and bi-manual co-ordination in children with hand–eye co-ordination problems. Nordisk Fysioterapi 3: 55–64

Sigmundsson H (2003) Perceptual deficits in clumsy children: inter- and intra-modal matching approach – a window into clumsy behaviour. Neural Plast 10: 27–38

Sigmundsson H, Whiting HTA (2002) Hand preference in children with developmental co-ordination disorders: cause and effect? Brain Cogn 49: 45–53

Sigmundsson H, Hopkins B (2004) Do 'clumsy' children have visual recognition problems? Child Care Health Dev 31: 155–158

Sigmundsson H, Ingvaldsen RP, Whiting HTA (1997a) Inter- and intra-sensory modality matching in children with hand–eye co-ordination problems. Exp Brain Res 114: 492–499

Sigmundsson H, Ingvaldsen RP, Whiting HTA (1997b) Inter- and intra-sensory modality matching in children with hand–eye co-ordination problems: exploring the developmental lag hypothesis. Dev Med Child Neurol 12: 790–796

Sigmundsson H, Whiting HTA, Ingvaldsen RP (1999a) Putting your foot in it! A window into clumsy behaviour. Behav Brain Res 102: 131–138

Sigmundsson H, Whiting HTA, Ingvaldsen RP (1999b) Proximal versus distal control in proprioceptively guided movements of motor-impaired children. Behav Brain Res 106: 47–54

Sigmundsson H, Hansen PC, Talcott JB (2003) Do 'clumsy children have visual deficits'. Behav Brain Res 139: 123–129

Smyth TR (1991) Abnormal clumsiness in children: a programming defect? Child Care Health Dev 17: 283–294

Smyth TR (1992) Impaired motor skill (clumsiness) in otherwise normal children: a review. Child Care Health Dev 18: 283–300

Smyth TR (1994) Clumsiness in children: a defect of kinaesthetic perception? Child Care Health Dev 20: 27–36

Sperry RW (1974) Lateral specialisation in the surgically separated hemispheres. In: Schmitt FO, Worden FG (eds) The neurosciences: third study program. MIT Press, Cambridge, pp 5–19

Stott DH (1966) A general test of motor impairment for children. Dev Med Child Neurol 8: 523–531

Søvik N, Mæland AF (1986) Children with motor problems ("clumsy children"). Scand J Educ Res 30: 39–53

Trevarthen C (1974) Cerebral embroylogy and the split brain. In: Kinsbourne M, Smith WL (eds) Hemispheric disconnection and cerebral function. Charles C Thomas, Springfield, pp 208–236

Walton JN, Ellis E, Court S (1962) Clumsy children: developmental apraxia and agnosia. Brain 85: 603–612

Yakolev PI, Lecours AR (1967) The myelogenetic cycles of regional maturationof the brain. In: Minkowski A (ed) Regional development of the brain in early life. Davis, Philadelphia

Zaidel E (1998) Sterognosis in the chronic split brain: hemispheric differences, ipsilateral control and sensory integration across the midline. Neuropsychologia 36: 1033–1047

Author's address: H. Sigmundsson, Research Group for Child Development, Department of Sociology and Political Science, Norwegian University of Science and Technology, Trondheim, Norway, e-mail: hermundur.sigmundsson@svt.ntnu.no

Tic disorders and obsessive compulsive disorder: where is the link?

V. Roessner, A. Becker, T. Banaschewski, and **A. Rothenberger**

Department of Child and Adolescent Psychiatry, University of Göttingen, Germany

Summary. Over the last years evidence on the overlap between tic-disorders (TD) and obsessive compulsive behavior/disorder (OCB/OCD) has increased. The main focus of research have been the phenomenological and epidemiological similarities and differences in samples of different age, primary diagnosis (TD vs. OCD) including the co-occurrence of both. Unfortunately, only a minority of studies included all three groups (TD, TD + OCD, OCD). Nevertheless, new insight concerning possible subtypes for both TD and OCD has been gained. While some authors concentrated on OCD with/without tics we will summarize the field of TD and OCB/OCD from the viewpoint of tics, since OCB plays an important role in patients with TD. Thereby we will not only sharpen the clinicans' awareness of known differences in phenomenology, epidemiology, genetics and neurobiology, aimed to improve their diagnoses and treatment but also highlight the gaps of knowledge and discuss possibilities for further research in this field.

Introduction

Since the 1980ies the clear distinction between tic-related and non-tic-related obsessive compulsive disorders (OCD) has received support from phenomenologic, family-genetic, psychopharmacologic, and neuroendocrine studies (Hanna et al., 1991; Leckman et al., 1994a; McDougle et al., 1994; Pauls et al., 1995).

Within the last years only four reviews have been published in journals on this issue. In 2001 Miguel et al. (2001) focused on OCD and its relationship to tics by presenting the findings of studies investigating phenomenological similarities, the patients subjective experiences associated with obsessive compulsive behavior (OCB) and the possible overlap of OCD + TD with early onset OCD and **P**ediatric **A**utoimmune **N**europsychiatric **D**isorders **A**ssociated with **S**treptococcus (PANDAS). Swerdlow (2001) chose a more balanced view concerning the weighting between tics and OCB. Two years later Miguel et al. (2003) summarized treatment strategies in OCD and their modifications when tics coexist. In the same year Banaschewski et al. (2003a) reviewed the basis of knowledge concerning compulsive phenomena in children with TD and attention deficit-hyperactive disorder (ADHD).

Since then some progress has been made. Based on the proposed tic-related subtype of OCD not only studies on phenomenological or epidemiological questions, but also more specific studies in genetics (Castillo et al., 2004; Hemmings et al., 2003; Urraca et al., 2004), psychopharmacology (Geller et al., 2003), behavioral therapy (Himle et al., 2003) and immunology (Hoekstra et al., 2004b; Murphy et al., 2004) have been done. Another way to approach the overlap between TD and OCD is subtyping both disorders (Calamari et al., 2004; Leckman, 2003). The development of such categories has made great progress and they have been used in non-phenomenological studies already, showing promising results, e.g. (Zhang et al., 2002).

Therefore an actual overview seems to be helpful in order to update the work of Miguel et al. (2001). While these authors started from OCB/OCD looking towards TD, our perspective will be the other way around, i.e. from TD towards OCB/OCD, which is a more common problem in childpsychiatric practice.

Phenomenology

The co-occurrence of tics and OCB is known in medicine since more than hundred years (Gilles de la Tourette, 1885). Over the times many different attempts to clarify the psychopathologic similarities and differences between tics and OCB have been undertaken (see Table 1). We will describe the state of the art concerning phenomenological aspects between the 'two poles of a spectrum' ranging from TD to OCD (Moll and Rothenberger, 1999) and take

Table 1. Clinical differences and similarities of tics (TIC) and obsessive-compulsive behavior (OCB)

TIC	OCB
Differences	
Sudden, short (jerking/twitching)	ritualistic
Fragmented movement	goal directed behavior
Premonitory urges (sensorimotor)	thoughts/images (cognitive-emotinal dissonance)
Not anxiety-related	mostly anxiety-related
Ego-syntonic	ego-dystonic
Involuntary (clustering sequence)	Voluntary (cycling)
Onset with elementary school (one peak)	onset after elementary school (two peaks)
Waxing and waning (from seconds to month)	little change over time
Also during sleep	never during sleep
Similarities	
Concentration decreases	concentration decreases
Expressed emotions increases	expressed emotions increases
Suppressible (shortterm)	suppressible (longterm)

a special look on sensory phenomena, supressibility, impulsivity and self injurious behavior. This might help clinicans to improve their diagnoses and treatment of patients of the comorbid group.

Tics are defined as sudden, involuntary, brief, rapid and non-rhythmic motor movements or vocal productions in the presence of unimpaired motor skills (Leckman, 2003). They cause purposeless and stereotyped motor actions (motor tics) or sounds (vocal tics) that are not suited to the circumstances, but can be sometimes confused with goal directed behavior (Leckman et al., 2001). Tics can be classified by their appearance, frequency, intensity and complexity (Leckman, 2003). Each of these factors has been included in clinical rating scales that have proven to be useful in monitoring tic severity (Goetz and Kompoliti, 2001; Leckman et al., 1989; Walkup et al., 1992).

One common feature for the classification of tics is the subdivision into motor vs. vocal tics (Leckman et al., 1989). Another dichotomous subdivision is based on the 'complexity' of tics: simple vs. complex tics. The first group involves only isolated muscles or sounds. The predominance of single patterns of simple tics varies between the studies and countries, but craniofacial tics are almost always much more common than truncal-axial tics (Chee and Sachdev, 1994). Anatomically, there is a rostro-caudal increase in age of onset of simple motor tics. The existence of similar changes of a special feature of OCB has not been investigated so far.

Tics can fluctuate from one part of the body to another. Interestingly it is sometimes reported by TS patients that there is a suggestibility of tics, i.e. old tics may transiently reappear (Robertson et al., 1999). Both could be observed in a similar way in OCB.

Since almost any voluntary movement or sound can emerge as a motor or vocal tic (Leckman et al., 1998a), this can lead to problems in differentiating between tics and OCB, particularly if complex motor tics exist (Evidente, 2000; Moll and Rothenberger, 1999; O'Connor, 2001).

Because all types of TD are more common in families with any TD, several studies have suggested that the various TD diagnoses exist along a single continuum defined by type and duration of the tics (Singer and Walkup, 1991) and that there is a genetic component in TD. The most commonly used diagnostic scheme, as outlined in the DSM-IV (American Psychiatric Association, 1994), divides TD into three main tic categories: transient TD (TTD), chronic motor or chronic vocal TD (CMTD or CVTD), and Tourette's disorder/syndrome (TS).

The most salient features of TTD are the fact that individuals can have both multiple motor and vocal tics and that the total duration of tic symptoms is no longer than 1 year.

CMTD or CVTD are defined by the presence of either motor or vocal tics lasting more than 1 year.

TS criteria require that both multiple motor and one or more vocal tics have been present during the illness, although not necessarily simultaneously. A course of more than 1 year without a tic-free period of more than 3 consecutive months has also to be present.

The latest model of possible subtyping of TD has been developed by Alsobrook and Pauls (2002). They have recently used an agglomerative hierarchical cluster and factor analysis to identify TS symptom dimensions for the future use in studies in the field of TD. Four symptom dimensions were identified, including: (1) aggressive phenomena (e.g., kicking, temper fits, argumentativeness), (2) purely motor and vocal tic symptoms, (3) compulsive phenomena (e.g., touching of others or objects, repetitive speech, throat clearing), and (4) tapping and absence of grunting.

The same approach to identify reliable and valid subtypes has been conducted in OCD, but the data are more widespread. In the different models nearly all based on Y-BOCS (for an overview see Table 1 in Calamari et al. (2004)) the number of subgroups ranges between 3 to 5 and in recent work greater support was found for a seven subgroup taxonomy. In all models three dimensions have been found: Contamination/Washing, Harming/Checking and Symmetry/Ordering.

But in both single disorders (TD or OCD) and especially in the comorbid group (TS + OCD) additional work remains to be done to test the suitability of these models of subtyping. Furthermore, it has to be clarified to which extent the dimension 'compulsive phenomena' of the model of Alsobrook and Pauls (2002) overlaps with the subtype 'tic-related OCD'.

Nevertheless, the potential for this effort remains high to elucidate etiological processes and improve treatment and research outcome (Calamari et al., 2004; Leckman, 2003).

Sensory phenomena

A sensory component preceding a motor tic has been described in numerous case reports and series (Bliss, 1980; Bullen and Hemsley, 1983; Cohen and Leckman, 1992; Kurlan et al., 1989; Lang, 1991; Leckman et al., 1994b; Miguel et al., 2000). In larger samples of patients with TD the frequency of various sensory phenomena ranges between 37% (Banaschewski et al., 2003b) to over 90% (Leckman et al., 1993). An increase during child development (not dependent on duration of TD) has been shown (Banaschewski et al., 2003b).

These premonitory sensations have been named as 'sensory tics', 'internal tics', 'an urge', an 'impulse', an 'itch', a 'pressure', and the 'just right' phenomenon (Cohen and Leckman, 1992; Kurlan et al., 1989; Leckman et al., 1993, 1994b).

The most common sensory phenomena in TD are unusual bodily sensations (tactile, muscular-skeletal or visceral) or an irresistible urge to move (Berardelli et al., 2003). Because patients often interpret their tics as 'intentional' movements directed to relieve 'involuntary' sensations that are so displeasing and connected with the urge to perform a motor action, that only the execution of a tic can abate the feeling of distress (Banaschewski et al., 2003b), they are often categorized as a sensorimotor disorder, unlike other involuntary hyperkinesias such as chorea, myoclonus, or tremor (Kwak et al., 2003; Scahill et al., 1995). Interestingly these sensations can even be located extra-corporeal ('phantom tics') (Karp and Hallett, 1996).

Frequently, the affected patients are unable to distinguish exactly between a 'unit' of premonitory sensations and the following tic or the appearance of the premonitory sensation as a long-lasting 'sensory' tic, which stops or decreases for a short period solely after executing the voluntary induced motor tic (Moll and Rothenberger, 1999).

This occurrence of tics in response to a local sensation or a more generalized urge can be assigned as a link to OCB (O'Connor, 2001), although in TD the series of tic movements may relieve bodily sensations without initiating a repetitive cycle. Hence, one should distinguish between the 'cycle of OCD' (O'Connor, 2001) and the 'clustering sequence of TD'.

The overlap between tics and OCB can be seen even in other criteria of obsessions by *DSM-IV.*

The existence of recurrent and persistent thoughts, impulses, or images, is experienced, at some time during the disturbance, as intrusive and inappropriate. The same estimation can be found in patients, who report that their tics are involuntary in parts and definitely not suited to the circumstances. Moreover, 36% of the subject who experience premonitory urges knew that the planned complex behaviors are dangerous or inappropriate, but they felt incapable of refraining from it (Cohen and Leckman, 1992).

Furthermore, like the obsessions that cause marked anxiety or distress, premonitory urges have been reported as distressing and painful by nearly all TD patients (Banaschewski et al., 2003b; Kurlan et al., 1989; Leckman et al., 1993), and from about the half as more bothersome than the tics themselves (Cohen and Leckman, 1992). But whereas tics have a sensorimotor character representing an urge, OCB must be seen as a cognitive-emotional dissonance with parallels to anxiety disorders (Comer et al., 2004).

Analog to the attempts to ignore or suppress such thoughts, impulses, or images or to neutralize them with some other thought or action, it has been proposed that motor tics are considered to be also tension reducing responses to a specific sensory stimulus (Banaschewski et al., 2003b; Evers and van de Wetering, 1994).

As the OCD patient recognizes that the obsessional thoughts, impulses, or images are a product of his or her own mind, some patients with TD sense their tics as not clearly involuntary in response to the premonitory phenomena.

More than two thirds of the patients with TD reported a heightened sensitivity to tactile, auditory, and/or visual stimuli (Cohen and Leckman, 1992) and a stimulus triggered performance of tics has been described commonly (Eapen et al., 1994; Leckman et al., 1998a).

Support for a strong association of sensory phenomena to the comorbid group (TD + OCD) comes also from a comparison between TS (n = 55) and TS + OCD (n = 16) with an increased rating in the latter group. There was no significant difference when comparing TS with TS + ADHD (n = 28) (own unpublished data).

Suppressibility

Another phenomenon in tics related to premonitory sensations is their suppressibility, i.e. the ability to exert some voluntary control over the tics for brief periods of time (Robertson et al., 1999). About 50% of patients with premonitory urges prior to motor and vocal tics thought the premonitory urges enhanced their ability to suppress tics (Cohen and Leckman, 1992). Like the premonitory urges the supressibility shows a nearly continuous increase from childhood to early adulthood (Banaschewski et al., 2003b).

Motor tics can be suppressed by an effort of will or concentration, but unfortunately this is often associated with an increase of inner tension and tics reappear or even rebound when the patient is relaxed (Jankovic, 1997; Leckman, 2003; Lees et al., 1984).

OCB can be also suppressed. Whereas the suppression of obsessions seem to lead to an increase or rebound (Tolin et al., 2002), the suppression of compulsions is used as a successful therapy (exposure and response prevention) (Hembree et al., 2003).

Published data for the comorbid group are missing, but we could observe a clearly higher ability to suppress tics in the comorbid group (n = 28) compared to the TS-only group (n = 78) (own unpublished data).

Waxing and waning

It is observed regularly that certain environmental factors as distressing events (family conflicts, financial problems, and problems associated with work), but also positive emotional arousal (e.g. birthdays, rewarding situations) or fatigue have been reported to exacerbate tics, whereas others like alcohol, relaxation or concentration on an enjoyable task may alleviate tics (Jankovic, 1997; Robertson, 2000; Silva et al., 1995). But in some patients who are able to suppress tics, relaxation may actually intensify their symptoms (Kuperman, 2002). Hence, there is a high variability of modulatory factors.

Periods of symptomatological remission in OCD may not only be spontaneous or induced by medication, but also related to favorable psychosocial factors (Perugi et al., 1998). About 50–70% of patients describe onsets preceded by stressful life events (Khanna et al., 1988; Neziroglu et al., 1992). Taken together, the role of life events or major stress in the occurrence of obsessions and compulsions is, like in TD, scarcely studied and no data exist for the comorbid group.

Regarding TD changes of symptoms during the natural course of the disorder could be attributed to three different time scales: (i) seconds, (ii) weeks to month, (iii) years. Unfortunately it is impossible to fully disentangle these confusions retrospectively. Nevertheless we will summarize the data of both groups (TD, OCD) and have to realize that there is little information about the comorbid group (de Groot, 1997; Lin et al., 2002).

Changes in seconds must be seen as tic specific because motor and vocal tics occur with variable frequency in bouts over the course of a day (Peterson and Leckman, 1998). A bout is defined by Leckman (2003) as a brief period of constant short intervals between each tic, typically 0.5–1.0 seconds.

Leckman proposed an 'extending' terminology: over the course of minutes to hours the bouts of tics themselves occur in bouts and that over the course of weeks to months, bouts-of-bouts-of-bouts-of-bouts of tics occur in bouts. This periodic higher-order combination of tic bouts is likely to be the basis of the well known 'waxing and waning' course of TD according to the before mentioned scale of weeks and month. Tics wax and wane in form, severity and frequency during their natural course (Leckman et al., 1998b; Peterson and Leckman, 1998; Robertson, 2000; Swedo et al., 1998). Less well known is the 'self-similarity' of these temporal patterns across the different time scales (Leckman, 2003; Leckman et al., 1998a; Swedo et al., 1998).

Based on several studies of the development of tics, according to a time window of years, many authors concluded (Bruun and Budman, 1992, 1997; Kuperman, 2002; Leckman et al., 1998b; Nee et al., 1980; Singer and Walkup, 1991; Goetz et al., 1992), that many patients reach complete remission during late adolescence or improve to the point that tics are relatively mild and do not cause severe impairment. The majority of the tics remitted by adolescence (Costello et al., 1996; Peterson et al., 2001a; Verhulst et al., 1997; Zohar et al., 1992).

In the first study using objective measurement roughly half of all TS patients experienced a significant diminution of symptoms in their early 20 s, but up to 90% had persistent, lifelong tics (Pappert et al., 2003). Interestingly, adult patients who considered themselves tic-free were often inaccurate in their self-assessment: 50% had objective evidence of tics (Pappert et al., 2003). There is consensus that tics with no decrease in adolescence might represent the subgroup with the highest rate of chronicity and severity. Interestingly, tic severity during childhood was not predictive of future course, but most patients with mild tics during late adolescence had mild tics during adulthood (Goetz et al., 1992).

Waxing and waning of symptoms could be found in OCD also, but nearly always without symptom changes in intervals of milliseconds to seconds. Some putative patients with a past history of OCD have demonstrated symptom-free periods of months or years (Ravizza et al., 1997), which seems to be longer than in TD.

Despite the limitations of the available data (for a short review see Mataix-Cols et al. (2002) and Steketee et al. (1999)), almost concurrently four categories of OCD course have been described in the DSM-IV (American-Psychiatric-Association, 1994). A replication of the pre-set prevalences given there by others has failed, probably because an estimate of the occurrence of the different courses is nearly impossible as appropriate criteria for their clear identification are still missing – a problem described by Ravizza et al. (1997).

Thus, the data reporting an episodic course range between 2% to 50% of patients affected, and waxing and waning of symptoms has been reported in up to 80% of the OCD patients (for a short review see Mataix-Cols et al. (2002) and Steketee et al. (1999)).

The sex ratio indicated that episodic OCD is more common in females, shows a higher age at onset of the disorder (Ravizza et al., 1991, 1997), more frequent lifetime comorbidity, bipolar-II and panic disorder (Perugi et al., 1998). Comparison of obsessions and compulsions did not show any difference between the two groups, with the exception of checking rituals, which were more frequently represented in patients with continuous course (Perugi et al., 1998). The chronic subtype presented more compulsive behavior and had a high rate of concomitant depressive symptomatology (Ravizza et al., 1991).

Concerning the time scale of years a meta-analysis of the long-term outcome of pediatric OCD revealed mean persistence rates of 41% for full OCD and 60% for full or subthreshold OCD what is lower than believed (Stewart et al., 2004). Unfortunately comorbid TD + OCD is not investigated in any of these studies.

Very few studies investigating the natural course of symptoms in a sample comorbid for TS and OCD have been published up to date (only time scale of weeks to month). Lin et al. (2002) included a small sample of 17 children and adolescents affected with TS and OCD. Their preliminary data showed that in children comorbid for TS and OCD fluctuations within these symptom domains showed a significant degree of synchronicity, but more detailed data are missing. De Groot et al. (1997) described after 5 years that tic symptoms have improved in 13% and OCB in 48%, but the findings are based on only 23 probands of the sample (n = 103, range 7–61 years).

The fact, that patients with an episodic course of OCD responded better to both clomipramine and fluoxetine compared with chronic patients (Ravizza et al., 1991), highlights once more the possible importance of subtyping not only OCD but also TD according to episodic vs. chronic courses of illness (Ravizza et al., 1997). Comparable data on TD is not available so far. In view of this an important and commonly underestimated problem could be discussed. A reduction of symptoms induced by medication does not justify speaking of an episodic course or vice versa (Perugi et al., 1998). The question of how to differentiate whether a spontaneous period of symptomatological remission or the start of a successful treatment caused a symptom-free interval, seems unresolved up to date in TD and OCD. Thus, especially the fluctuations of tics and OCB over time are important for clincans to decide about upon starting interventions and rate its effects correctly (Leckman, 2003; Perugi et al., 1998; Roessner et al., 2004).

Several efforts for identifying underlying factors of tic symptom exacerbations have been undertaken so far (Leckman, 2002; Lin et al., 2002; Singer et al., 2000). It has been found that the period of greatest tic fluctuation was observed in patients between the ages of 10 to 12 years of age (Leckman, 2002; Lin et al., 2002), a time when the tics are most severe in many children (Leckman et al., 1998b). In OCB/OCD such a peak could be seen around 12–16 years and in the early twenties. But no causal relationship has been identified.

In both disorders previous efforts to identify predictors of the course of the symptoms suggested relatively few consistent predictors among demographic variables. Findings regarding the effects of comorbid conditions are uncertain, probably because sample sizes have been too small to detect the effects even of relatively infrequent disorders (Leckman, 2003; Steketee et al., 1999) and the unresolved questions of the terms and definitions (Keck et al., 1998), especially in OCD (Ravizza et al., 1997). Thus, longer longitudinal studies involving larger samples of children and adults with OCD are needed to further understand the longer-term course of OCB (Mataix-Cols et al., 2002) and tics, as well as the relationship between childhood and adulthood forms of the disorders.

Self injurious behavior

Self injurious behavior occurs with varying frequency in movement disorders (Mathews et al., 2004), most notably in TS (Robertson et al., 1989) when OCD is associated. Therefore we will report the data on SIB in TS and TS + OCB/OCD. To our knowledge there is no study on SIB in OCD. Only OCB expressed by hair-pulling and skin-picking has been defined as SIB.

Self injurious behavior is observed in 4% to 60% of patients with TS, although frequency varies depending on the definition of self injury (Cath et al., 2001a; Eisenhauer and Woody, 1987; Freeman et al., 2000; Mathews et al., 2004; Robertson et al., 1989). Different forms of self injurious behavior have been reported in individuals with TS, including compulsive head banging, eye damage from self poking, skin picking, self hitting, filing of the teeth and lip and other self biting (for a review see Robertson et al. (1989)).

Severe self injurious behavior has been observed in 4% of the patients with TS of all ages (Mathews et al., 2004). Severe long lasting or incurable physical damage, e.g. blindness from retinal detachment can also occur in a small minority of adolescent and adult cases secondary to severe self-injurous tics (Leckman, 2003).

Freeman et al. (2000) demonstrated self injurious behavior in 14% of 3500 individuals with TS collected from all over the world. Individuals who had TS plus at least one other psychiatric comorbidity had a fourfold increase in self injurious behavior, and there was a positive linear relationship between the number of psychiatric comorbidities and the presence of self injurious behavior. In this sample, the presence of OCD but not ADHD was highly correlated with self injurious behavior (Freeman et al., 2000).

A similar pattern of correlation, namely between self injurious behavior and severity of tic symptoms as well as high levels of obsessionality and hostility has been measured using a number of subjective rating scales (Robertson and Gourdie, 1990; Robertson et al., 1989). Examining a group comorbid for TS and OCD Cath et al. (2000) found significantly more severe and more SIB than in the OCD group. One case report focused on the different treatment options of severe SIB in coexisting TS and OCD (Hood et al., 2004). Recently, Mathews et al. (2004) could show a dichotomy in correlation: for mild/moderate self injurious behavior in TS the most important predictor variables appeared to be related to OCD symptoms such as the presence of aggressive obsessions or violent or aggressive compulsions, the presence of the diagnosis of an OCD and the sum of the obsessions. On the other hand, severe self injurious behavior in TS was correlated with variables related to affect or impulse control mechanisms; in particular, with the presence of episodic rages and risk taking behavior. The authors concluded that mild/moderate and severe self injurious behavior in TS may represent different phenomena, what has some implications for differentiation in clinical management of these symptoms.

Impulsivity

A deficit in impulse control mechanisms has not exclusively been found in TS patients with severe self injurious behavior. Disruptive behaviors such as aggression, anger control problems, rage attacks, and noncompliance has been observed also in clinical samples of children with TS (Budman et al., 1998, 2000; Freeman et al., 2000; Rosenberg et al., 1995; Stephens and Sandor, 1999; Stokes et al., 1991; Sukhodolsky et al., 2003), in community surveys (Stefl, 1984) and community samples (Kadesjo and Gillberg, 2000; Peterson et al., 2001a).

Most authors suggested that the risk for aggressive and delinquent behavior in children with TS is posed largely by the presence of ADHD (Sukhodolsky et al., 2003) or ADHD + OCD (Budman et al., 1998; Stephens and Sandor, 1999). Freeman (2000) reported anger control problems in patients with TS solely in 10%, with TS comorbid for ADHD-only in 25%, comorbid for OCD-only in 16% and comorbid for ADHD + OCD in 40%. Similar findings have been described by Banaschewski et al. (2003a): the comorbid group showed higher rates of impulsive and aggressive behaviors.

This is in accordance with the proposal to classify probands with OCD into impulsive and non-impulsive subgroups. Thus, OCD patients may experience interne anger, and at least a subset of OCD patients have been documented to have difficulties in controlling anger (Hoehn-Saric and Barksdale, 1983). Stein et al. (1994) found that impulsivity scores correlated positively with severity of OCD symptoms. During successful treatment of OCD there is a reduction in impulsivity and anger (Farid, 1986; Lopez-Ibor, 1990).

Tic-related OCD patients have a higher rate of distressing violent or aggressive thoughts or images, or worries about symmetry and exactness and less contamination obsessions and cleaning compulsions (see Table 2) (Baer, 1994; de Groot et al., 1994; George et al., 1993; Holzer et al., 1994; Leckman et al., 1994a; Swerdlow et al., 1999; Moll et al., 2000).

Table 2. Expression of OCB features; clinical estimation on the basis of the literature and practical experiences. There is a clear weight for cognitive-emotional driven behavior in OCD, while TD reflect merely sensorimotor aspects

OCB feature	OCD	TD
Cleanness	+++	(+)
Sexuality	+++	(+)
Religion	+++	(+)
Controlling	+++	(+)
Counting	+++	+
Symmetry	++	+++
Touching/rubbing	+	++
Tipping/breaking	(+)	+++
Repetitions	++	++
Ordering	++	(+)
Hoarding	+	(+)
Selfinjuries	+	++
Rituals	+(+)	++
Obsessions	+++	(+)
Associated fears	+++	+

+ = low, ++ = intermediate, +++ = high

The fact that impulsivity correlated positively with aggressive and sexual OCD symptoms, but negatively with cleaning and checking symptoms (Stein et al., 1994), could be regarded as another distinguishing feature and hint for the existence of a tic-related OCD subtype.

To which extent the coexistence of aggression in TS and OCD may be based on possible basal ganglia pathology has been discussed by Yaryura-Tobias (2003).

Epidemiology

Besides the similarities in phenomenology of tics and OCB their coexistence has been the most obvious and frequently studied topic. First, data on TD-only and thereafter for the comorbid group will be presented.

TD

TD are found in all cultures, countries, and racial groups (Khalifa and von Knorring, 2003). The prevalence for TD ranges from 1% to 30%, with the majority of studies finding that about 10% of youngsters have tics (for an overview see Table 1 in Lanzi et al. (2004) and Khalifa and von Knorring (2003); Peterson et al. (2001a); Wang and Kuo (2003)). Estimates of prevalence vary across clinical and field samples, because of differences in diagnostic criteria and thresholds (Lanzi et al., 2004; Rothenberger et al., 2005). Transient tics are more common (4%–24%) (Comings et al., 1990; Nomoto and Machiyama, 1990; Scahill et al., 2001; Wang and Kuo, 2003) than chronic TD with a prevalence of 1% to 5% (Khalifa and von Knorring, 2003; Scahill et al., 2001; Zohar et al., 1992). Tics may be present lifelong in some persons (Coffey et al., 2000).

The generally accepted prevalence for TS is about 0.5%–1.0% (Costello et al., 1996; Hornse et al., 2001; Kadesjo and Gillberg, 2000; Khalifa and von Knorring, 2003; Mason et al., 1998; Nomoto and Machiyama, 1990; Peterson et al., 2001a; Verhulst et al., 1997; Wang and Kuo, 2003), although studies over the last twenty years vary between about 0.01%–3.0% (Bruun, 1984; Scahill, 2001). The morbid risk for TS among relatives range between 9.8% and 15% across all studies and the rate of other tics ranges between 15% and 20% (Pauls, 2003).

There is considerable variation in the ratio of females to males (Bruun, 1984; Bruun and Budman, 1997; Chang et al., 2004; Freeman et al., 2000; Khalifa and von Knorring, 2003; Leckman et al., 1998b; Robertson, 1989), ranging from 1:10 (Comings et al., 1990) to 1:2 (Apter et al., 1993; Costello et al., 1996).

TD and OCD

Rates of OCB/OCD in TS patients usually range between 20–60% (Apter et al., 1993; Cardona et al., 2004; Chang et al., 2004; Comings and Comings, 1985; Frankel et al., 1986; Grad et al., 1987; Leckman et al., 1994b; Robertson et al., 1988).

There are also comorbid tics in OCD patients (6%–30%) (Bhattacharyya et al., 2004; Diniz et al., 2004; Grados et al., 2001; Holzer et al., 1994; Leonard et al., 1992).

Family studies give additional support for this relationship showing not only increased rates of tics in OCD patients and their relatives (Grados et al., 2001; Leonard et al., 1992; Nestadt et al., 2003; Pauls et al., 1995) but also increased rates (2–5 times higher) of OCD among family members of patients with TS, regardless of whether the proband had comorbid OCD (Comings and Comings, 1987; Eapen et al., 1993; Hebebrand et al., 1997; Pauls et al., 1991b). These findings strengthen the idea of an association between at least some forms of TD and OCD and might therefore be a variant expression of the same unknown etiologic factors (Cath et al., 2001b; Pauls et al., 1995).

Lower rates of OCD in subjects with tics are probably caused by the restriction of the sample to children (obsessive thoughts and compulsive rituals first appear several years after the onset of motor tics (Kuperman, 2002; Kurlan et al., 2002)). Nevertheless the distinction between tic-related and non-tic-related OCD is also supported by data indicating an earlier age of onset for tic-related OCD (de Groot et al., 1994; Leonard et al., 1992; Mataix-Cols et al., 1999). Nearly 60% of children and adolescents with OCD will develop tics at some point in their lives (Leonard et al., 1992).

Tic-related OCD occurs more often in males than in females (George et al., 1993; Leckman et al., 1994a; Leonard et al., 1992; Mataix-Cols et al., 1999).

Genetics

Although genetic factors play an important role in both TD and OCD, the phenotype may be variable and other moderating variables can be assumed (for a review see Grados et al. (2003); Pauls (2003)). For more promising findings studies of subgroups like tic-related OCD should be advanced.

TD

It has been reported that a pattern of vertical transmission of TS fitted best to a mode of inheritance involving a single autosomal dominant locus with varying penetrance (Devor, 1984; Eapen et al., 1993; Pauls et al., 1991a; Pauls and Leckman, 1986), while more recent studies have indicated that the genetic transmission is probably more complex (Hanna et al., 1999; Hasstedt et al., 1995; Kurlan et al., 1994; Lichter et al., 1995; Seuchter et al., 2000; Walkup et al., 1996; Zhang et al., 2002).

A number of candidate loci have been examined for TS and all together the results are generally negative. Only for the DRD4 positive results have been published (Diaz-Anzaldua et al., 2004; Grice et al., 1996).

Studies on candidate regions have been undertaken with mixed results; some regions with preliminary but unconfirmed hints of possible linkage have been proposed on the chromosomes 3, 7, 8, 18 (for a review see Pauls (2003)).

Although there is a clear involvement of genetic factors in TS, the non-100% concordance rates for TS in monozygotic twins (Price et al., 1985) also point to the involvement of nongenetic elements like adverse prenatal events (Hyde et al., 1992; Leckman et al., 1990). Further, in a small subgroup PANDAS may play a role (Hoekstra et al., 2004a).

TD and OCD

There is increasing evidence towards the involvement of the dopaminergic and serotonergic systems in the development of OCD and genetic studies have found that at least a subgroup of OCD patients is genetically related to TS (Pauls et al., 1991b, 1995; Pauls and Leckman, 1986). Additionally, the existence of a subtype of early-onset OCD, that appears to exhibit distinct clinical features and is associated with greater familial loading, seems to be confirmed step by step (for a review see Miguel et al. (2001)).

Based on this subtype Hemmings et al. (2003) found an increased frequency of tics, trichotillomania and TS in an OCD sample and showed significant results when the allelic distributions of genetic variants in the dopamine receptor type 4 gene (DRD4) were analyzed. The result seems to support previous hypothesis that the dopaminergic systems may be relevant to the mediation of early-onset OCD and also to the possible overlap of early-onset OCD and tic-related OCD. Cruz et al. (1997) could show that patients with OCD and comorbid TD (91%) compared to those with OCD-only (48%) showed at least one copy of the 7-fold variant of the 48 base-pair repeats (VNTR) in the DRD4. This finding was replicated onc ycar latcr by the same research group (48% OCD + TD vs. 9% OCD) (Nicolini et al., 1998), but it was not controlled for comorbid ADHD, which shows a high association to DRD4-7.

Interestingly only the results from one single candidate gene study in TS (Grice et al., 1996) were consistent with an apparent association between the DRD4 locus and TS. Unfortunately, Hebebrand et al. (1997) were unable to replicate the association using a family-based paradigm and Barr et al. (1996) did not find any evidence for linkage in a sample of Canadian families using three different polymorphisms in the DRD4 locus. In OCD also significant differences in allele frequencies were found between patients and controls for the 48-base-pair repeat in the DRD4 gene (Billett et al., 1998). A further attempt to replicate the association using the 2 allele for the 48 bp repeat polymorphism of the DRD4 gene failed (Millet et al., 2003).

Concerning a genetic role for the involvement of the serotonergic system in OCD, a statistically significant preferential transmission of the G861C polymorphism of the 5 HT1Dbeta gene was found. These preliminary results suggested that the G861C polymorphism of 5 HT1Dbeta gene could be a marker of tic-related OCD and should be confirmed further in larger samples (Castillo et al., 2004).

Between μ-opioid receptor (MOR) gene and OCD no significant association has been found. However, the possibility that MOR could be related to OCD patients with tics can not be ruled out definitely and should be replicated in further family-based association studies (Urraca et al., 2004).

Furthermore, data from one specific study strongly suggested that coding variations of IMMP2L and NrCAM do not play a major role in TS and OCD etiology. These results also delineate the screening of additional candidate genes in the 7q31 region (Chabane et al., 2004).

In the investigation of another OCD subtype, the hoarding phenotype (a component of OCD) a reanalysis of the TS Association (TSA) sib pair sample using a recursive partitioning analytic technique found evidence for hoarding symptoms related to chromosomes 4, 5, and 17 (Zhang et al., 2002).

In conclusion the value of auxiliary studies is supported, which utilize (1) phenotypic subtyping (using comorbid conditions) and (2) endophenotyping based on brain mechanisms underlying OCD (functional brain imaging and neuropsychological measures) in order to delineate the complex genetics of this severe and debilitating psychiatric disorder (Grados et al., 2003; Hemmings et al., 2003).

Treatment

The treatment options for patients with OCD and coexisting tics have been reviewed by Miguel et al. (2003). Further, some progress of evaluating the efficacy of psychotherapeutic treatment techniques that are used in both TD and OCD has been reported (Hembree et al., 2003; Tolin et al., 2004; Verdellen et al., 2004; Wilhelm et al., 2003; Woods et al., 2003). We will present this progress and extend the information given by Miguel et al. (2003).

Medication

If impairment interferes with daily activities and leads to psychosocial suffering, medication remains the cornerstone of therapy especially in tics, and therapy should be individualized to treat the most distressing symptom(s) (Rothenberger and Banaschewski, 2004).

In treatment of TD worldwide clonidine and (from the group of novel antipsychotics) risperidone show the broadest empirical basis while in Europe benzamides have a good empirical clinical background (for a review see Marcus and Kurlan (2001), Roessner et al. (2004), Rothenberger and Banaschewski (2004)). In OCD SSRIs are the first line in pharmacological treatment (for a review see Dougherty et al. (2004)). However, because some patients do not respond to SSRIs monotherapy, various augmentation strategies are currently recommended.

In OCD patients with tics fluoxetine showed in one study a modest improvement of tics (Kurlan et al., 1993) whereas in the other no effect on tics had been observed (Scahill et al., 1997). In another study with fluvoxamine monotherapy clinical improvement occurred less often in the OCD + tics group compared to the OCD-only group. After the addition of a neuroleptic the vast majority of the patients refractory to SSRI treatment alone responded (McDougle et al., 1993, 1994). In their review Miguel at al. (2003) added results of an unpublished, systematic, blind study in 41 OCD patients treated for 14 weeks with clomipramine which did not confirm the presence of tics or TS as predictive of a poor response. Furthermore, they reported unpublished results of a nonsystematic evaluation of another sample (30 OCD, 50% with current or past chronic tics) that did not reveal tics as predictors of poor treatment response in a longer follow-up assessment.

In addition to the benefical effect on tic symptoms of risperidone (for a review see Roessner et al. (2004)), this drug led to significant improvement of coexisting OCB. Prior investigators have reported this finding in open-label studies (Bruun and Budman, 1996; Giakas, 1995; Lombroso et al., 1995). In a controlled study, the 23 TS adolescent and adult patients with comorbid OCD showed improvement on both risperidone and pimozide according to reduced Y-BOCS scores. However the change from baseline was significant only for risperidone (Bruggeman et al., 2001).

In a double-blind study to evaluate the efficacy and tolerability of risperidone in comparison with clonidine in the treatment of children and adolescents with TS the 20 patients with coexisting OCD showed no differences between the risperidone and clonidine groups concerning their baseline to endpoint improvements on the used OCD-scale (Gaffney et al., 2002).

In contrast olanzapine had no significant influence on OCB (Budman et al., 2001). However olanzapine has shown good property to reduce aggressions and tics in children with TS (Stephens et al., 2004).

These preliminary data from small sample sizes suggest that risperidone may have good efficacy for OCB in TS, while the findings of olanzapine and other neuroleptics warrant further investigation.

Behavioral psychotherapy

In TD various specific psychological therapies such as relaxation therapy, habit reduction techniques and habit reversal therapy for the tics have been described (Faridi and Suchowersky, 2003). Cognitive-behavior therapy (CBT) is the psychological treatment of choice in OCD (Van Noppen et al., 1997), mainly through the techniques of exposure and response prevention (ERP).

Because both TS and OCD are usually seen as a chronic and disabling disorder, the current treatments, most of the time, only alleviate the symptoms but do not cure. Therefore, education of the family, child, and school personnel regarding the impairing and involuntary character, natural course, prognosis and treatment is essential as well as help to contact family and patient organizations. Because the family dynamics often may have great modulating influence family intervention should be considered in some cases (Calvocoressi et al., 1995).

No studies exist that test the different effects of cognitive-behavioral therapy (CBT), the psychological treatment of choice in OCD (Franklin et al., 1998; March et al., 2001; Piacentini et al., 2002) for tic-related vs. non-tic-related OCD. At least two anecdotal reports suggest that tic-related OCD may not respond as well to CBT as does non-tic-related OCD (King et al., 1998; Leckman et al., 2000). This observation may be in part due to symptom profile differences between tic-related and non-tic-related OCD, as noted above (see Table 2). Contamination/washing and doubting/checking symptoms are less common in tic-related OCD but have been shown to respond better to CBT (Buchanan et al., 1996; Drummond, 1993).

But recently ERP as well as habit reversal (HR) resulted in statistically significant improvements of TS symptoms (Verdellen et al., 2004). A tendency in favor of ERP was found on the YGTSS.

Alternatives in treatment refractory cases

In treatment refractory cases several methods have been used experimentally.

In stereotactic lesioning thalamic and infrathalamic targets are chosen for alleviating tics whereas cingulotomy and leucotomy may improve OCB (Berardelli et al., 2003).

Over the last decade, deep brain stimulation (DBS) has shown superiority over previous lesioning procedures, particularly in movement disorders like TS (Visser-Vandewalle et al., 2004). In view of the psychiatric and cognitive effects seen in neurosurgery it seems to be promising to study DBS in the treatment of refractory psychiatric disease. The few published studies on DBS for OCD suggest that this can be done safely with placing the electrode in the nucleus accumbens (Tass et al., 2003). Efficacy data are still uncertain, but initial data are promising (Kopell et al., 2004). In addition the question of its use in comorbid TS and OCD has to be clarified.

In a case report a 39-year-old female patient with chronic TS and OCD was presented whose symptomatology resolved fairly rapidly after a course of nine electroconvulsive treatments. Under outpatient ECT sessions remission of both disorders has been maintained successfully for more than a year (Strassnig et al., 2004). This is in line with reports of successful treatment with ECT for patients with comorbid depression and TD (Rapoport et al., 1998; Swerdlow et al., 1990) but not with unsuccessful ECT in TS (Guttmacher and Cretella, 1988). Recently, Triverdi et al. (Trivedi et al., 2003) reported successful ECT in a TS type with catatonia. Further, ECT also has been used with mixed success in refractory OCD (Casey and Davis, 1994; Maletzky et al., 1994; Mellman and Gorman, 1984) and for patients with comorbid depression and OCD (Thomas and Kellner, 2003).

Using repetitive transcranial magnetic stimulation (rTMS) tic symptoms in 8 adults improved significantly over the 5 days of the study with minimal side effects (Chae et al., 2004). In OCD none or at most a proportion (about one quarter) of patients with resistant OCD regarded to respond to rTMS (Sachdev et al., 2001). But further studies using rTMS in TS as well in OCD with balanced parallel designs have to test this observed benefit (for a review in OCD see Martin et al. (2003)).

Neurobiology

The similarities in the area of neurobiology seem to be far less obvious and directly linked than in the other fields of research. Additionally, few studies focusing on comorbidity of TD + OCD have been performed. For TS a detailed review on its neurobiology and neuroimmunology has been published recently (Hoekstra et al., 2004a). The latter topic seems to be important concerning the overlap of TS and OCD.

Due to the phenomenology and natural history of TD, cortico-striato-thalamo-cortical (CSTC) circuits have been suggested to be involved in TD (Leckman et al., 1997) and OCD (Rauch et al., 2001). At least five functionally and anatomically distinct CSTC circuits have been proposed, which subserve motor, sensorimotor, oculomotor, cognitive, and limbic processes (for a review see Mink (2001), Tekin and Cummings (2002)).

A failure to inhibit specific CSTC circuit subsets has been hypothesized to be involved in tics and related disorders, and may be directly linked to specific types of tics, given the somatotopical organization of these CSTC circuits. For example, facial tics could be associated with a failure of inhibition of CSTC circuits that include the ventromedian areas of the caudate and putamen and that receive topographical projections from the orofacial regions of the (pre)motor cortex, whereas the limbic circuit may be associated with vocalizations, comorbid OCD and externalizing behavior problems (Mink, 2001; Tekin and Cummings, 2002). Neuropsychological data provided further evidence for a substantial impairment of the frontal-striatal-thalamic-frontal circuit in TD + OCD patients (Müller et al., 2003), but confounding problems with comorbid ADHD are not ruled out.

The possible involvement of the basal ganglia and related cortical structures in TD (Peterson et al., 2001b, 2003), OCD (Calabrese et al., 1993) and both TD and OCD (Saba et al., 1998) is supported by MRI studies. Basal ganglia volumes were not found to correlate significantly with the severity of tics (Peterson et al., 2003).

Previous functional imaging studies of subjects with TS have shown hypoperfusion of striatal and frontal areas (for a review see Peterson (2001c)), whereas studies of patients with primary OCD have shown hyperperfusion of similar areas (for a review see Saxena and Rauch (2000)). In a family study it could be shown that regional cerebral blood flow patterns in OCD-only patients from families affected by TS are comparable to their relatives with TS-only (Moriarty et al., 1997). This supports the assumption that the genetic background determines this neurobiological pattern and one might speculate that different pathways depending on the family history could lead to a similar TS + OCD phenotype.

Studies using TMS techniques evaluating motor networks showed that TS + OCD seems to be different from TS-only (Greenberg et al., 2000; Ziemann et al., 1997).

In the field of neurotransmitters the relationship between TD and OCD suggests that the serotonergic system is involved when OCB is diagnosed either alone or in combination with TD, while TD-only is merely related to the dopaminergic system.

It has been observed that a subgroup of children with TD and/or OCD have the onset and subsequent exacerbations of their symptoms following infections with group A beta-hemolytic streptococci (GABHS). Thus, a subgroup of childhood-onset TD and OCD with a postinfectious autoimmune-mediated etiology has been named PANDAS (**p**ediatric **a**utoimmune **n**europsychiatric **d**isorders **a**ssociated with **s**treptococcal infections) (Swedo et al., 1998). In view of the known etiology immunomodulatory therapies such as plasma exchange and intravenous immunoglobulins have shown some improvement of both tics and OCB (Murphy and Pichichero, 2002; Snider and Swedo, 2003). However, recently ELISA measurements of anti-basal ganglia antibodies did not differentiate between PANDAS and controls, suggesting a lack of major antibody changes in this disorder (Singer et al., 2004) which is in contrast to the findings of Church et al. (2004). Hence, this is still a field of controversial research (Kurlan, 2004; Luo et al., 2004; Martino et al., 2004).

Recently, Hounie et al. (2004) reported elevated rates of OCD, TD and other obsessive-compulsive spectrum disorders in patients with rheumatic fever (RF) in presence or absence of Sydenham's chorea. They suggested that these findings raise the possibility that some cases of PANDAS may be part of the RF spectrum manifestations.

Conclusions

Taken together, several links between TD and OCB can be detected but there remain many gaps for a better understanding. Further research may clarify, which of the four symptom dimensions of TD proposed by Alsobrook and Pauls (2002) might be related more closely with OCB/OCD. Actually category 3 'compulsive phenomena' seems to be one candidate regarding the findings that 70–80% of tic-related OCD patients have compulsions to touch, tap or rub items compared to only 5–25% of non-tic-related OCD patients (George et al., 1993; Leckman et al., 1994b). Category 1 'aggressive phenomena' would be interesting because of the higher rate of violent or aggressive thoughts or images in tic-related OCD patients (Baer, 1994; de Groot et al., 1994; George et al., 1993; Holzer et al., 1994; Leckman et al., 1994a).

Assuming that a specific limbic CSTC circuit may be associated with vocalizations, comorbid OCD and externalizing behavior problems (Mink, 2001; Tekin and Cummings, 2002) and the fact that a trend towards more compulsions than obsessions in the existence of higher impulsivity has been found (Stein et al., 1994) it has to be examined if phenotypic subgroups could be established and related to genetic or neurobiological markers. Moreover sensorimotor phenomena as a common feature of TS, may be helpful to investigate a subpopulation of TS patients with OCB/OCD, thereby testing the hypothesis of Chee et al. (1997) that sensorimotor phenomena represent the subjectively experienced component of neural dysfunction below the threshold for motor and vocal tic production. Contrarily, it could be hypothesized, that they might be merely a feature of underlying OCB.

Finally, the relationship between early-onset OCD and tic-related OCD has to be clarified. It has been proposed that the age at onset of OCD symptoms is an important feature in distinguishing OCD subgroups (Geller et al., 1998; Miguel et al., 1997; Rosario-Campos et al., 2001) and it has been reported that early-onset OCD patients have specific clinical correlates (Geller et al., 1998) with higher association with TD (Rosario-Campos et al., 2001), are more frequently found in males (Zohar et al., 1997), and have an increased familial loading for OCD (Nestadt et al., 2000; Pauls et al., 1995; Ravizza et al., 1997). However, there have been reports that the duration of illness might affect the OCD presentation as well (Ravizza et al., 1995, 1997). Another topic needs our attention because of both basic knowledge and therapeutic implications. Whereas TD and possibly trichotillomania may arise as a result of common etiologic 'sensorimotor' pathways, depressive disorders, in contrast, may be a secondary complication of the 'emotional-cognitive dissonance' OCD (Diniz et al., 2004).

In sum, the relationship between TD and OCD remains an important and exciting field of research and clinics. The link between both disorders reflects a variable, complex and dynamic interaction along the lifespan.

References

Alsobrook JP 2nd, Pauls DL (2002) A factor analysis of tic symptoms in Gilles de la Tourette's syndrome. Am J Psychiatry 159: 291–296

American Psychiatric Association (1994) Diagnostic and statistical manual of mental disorders. American Psychiatric Association, Washington

Apter A, Pauls DL, Bleich A, Zohar AH, Kron S, Ratzoni G, Dycian A, Kotler M, Weizman A, Gadot N, et al. (1993) An epidemiologic study of Gilles de la Tourette's syndrome in Israel. Arch Gen Psychiatry 50: 734–738

Azrin NH, Nunn RG (1973) Habit-reversal: a method of eliminating nervous habits and tics. Behav Res Ther 11: 619–628

Baer L (1994) Factor analysis of symptom subtypes of obsessive compulsive disorder and their relation to personality and tic disorders. J Clin Psychiatry 55 [Suppl]: 18–23

Banaschewski T, Siniatchkin M, Uebel H, Rothenberger A (2003a) [Compulsive phenomena in children with tic disorder and attention deficit-hyperactive disorder]. Z Kinder Jugendpsychiatr Psychother 31: 203–211

Banaschewski T, Woerner W, Rothenberger A (2003b) Premonitory sensory phenomena and suppressibility of tics in Tourette syndrome: developmental aspects in children and adolescents. Dev Med Child Neurol 45: 700–703

Barr CL, Wigg KG, Sandor P (1999) Catechol-O-methyltransferase and Gilles de la Tourette syndrome. Mol Psychiatry 4: 492–495

Barr CL, Wigg KG, Zovko E, Sandor P, Tsui LC (1996) No evidence for a major gene effect of the dopamine D4 receptor gene in the susceptibility to Gilles de la Tourette syndrome in five Canadian families. Am J Med Genet 67: 301–305

Barr CL, Wigg KG, Zovko E, Sandor P, Tsui LC (1997) Linkage study of the dopamine D5 receptor gene and Gilles de la Tourette syndrome. Am J Med Genet 74: 58–61

Berardelli A, Curra A, Fabbrini G, Gilio F, Manfredi M (2003) Pathophysiology of tics and Tourette syndrome. J Neurol 250: 781–787

Bhattacharyya S, Reddy YCJ, Khanna S, Prasanna CLN (2004) Is the genetic pool of OCD and tic disorder absent in India? In: Abstracts XIIth World Congress of Psychiatric Genetics. Am J Med Genet Part B: Neuropsychiatr Genet 130B: 68

Billett EA, Richter MA, Sam F, Swinson RP, Dai XY, King N, Badri F, Sasaki T, Buchanan JA, Kennedy JL (1998) Investigation of dopamine system genes in obsessive-compulsive disorder. Psychiatr Genet 8: 163–169

Bliss J (1980) Sensory experiences of Gilles de la Tourette syndrome. Arch Gen Psychiatry 37: 1343–1347

Brett PM, Curtis D, Robertson MM, Gurling HM (1995) The genetic susceptibility to Gilles de la Tourette syndrome in a large multiple affected British kindred: linkage analysis excludes a role for the genes coding for dopamine D1, D2, D3, D4, D5 receptors, dopamine beta hydroxylase, tyrosinase, and tyrosine hydroxylase. Biol Psychiatry 37: 533–540

Brett PM, Curtis D, Robertson MM, Gurling HM (1997) Neuroreceptor subunit genes and the genetic susceptibility to Gilles de la Tourette syndrome. Biol Psychiatry 42: 941–947

Bruggeman R, van der Linden C, Buitelaar JK, Gericke GS, Hawkridge SM, Temlett JA (2001) Risperidone versus pimozide in Tourette's disorder: a comparative double-blind parallel-group study. J Clin Psychiatry 62: 50–56

Bruun RD (1984) Gilles de la Tourette's syndrome. An overview of clinical experience. J Am Acad Child Psychiatry 23: 126–133

Bruun RD, Budman CL (1992) The natural history of Tourette syndrome. Adv Neurol 58: 1–6

Bruun RD, Budman CL (1996) Risperidone as a treatment for Tourette's syndrome. J Clin Psychiatry 57: 29–31

Bruun RD, Budman CL (1997) The course and prognosis of Tourette syndrome. Neurol Clin 15: 291–298

Buchanan AW, Meng KS, Marks IM (1996) What predicts improvement and compliance during the behavioral treatment of obsessive compulsive disorder? Anxiety 2: 22–27

Budman CL, Bruun RD, Park KS, Lesser M, Olson M (2000) Explosive outbursts in children with Tourette's disorder. J Am Acad Child Adolesc Psychiatry 39: 1270–1276

Budman CL, Bruun RD, Park KS, Olson ME (1998) Rage attacks in children and adolescents with Tourette's disorder: a pilot study. J Clin Psychiatry 59: 576–580

Budman CL, Gayer A, Lesser M, Shi Q, Bruun RD (2001) An open-label study of the treatment efficacy of olanzapine for Tourette's disorder. J Clin Psychiatry 62: 290–294

Bullen JG, Hemsley DR (1983) Sensory experience as a trigger in Gilles de la Tourette's syndrome. J Behav Ther Exp Psychiatry 14: 197–201

Calabrese G, Colombo C, Bonfanti A, Scotti G, Scarone S (1993) Caudate nucleus abnormalities in obsessive-compulsive disorder: measurements of MRI signal intensity. Psychiatry Res 50: 89–92

Calamari JE, Wiegartz PS, Riemann BC, Cohen RJ, Greer A, Jacobi DM, Jahn SC, Carmin C (2004) Obsessive-compulsive disorder subtypes: an attempted replication and extension of a symptom-based taxonomy. Behav Res Ther 42: 647–670

Calvocoressi L, Lewis B, Harris M, Trufan SJ, Goodman WK, McDougle CJ, Price LH (1995) Family accommodation in obsessive-compulsive disorder. Am J Psychiatry 152: 441–443

Cardona F, Romano A, Bollea L, Chiarotti F (2004) Psychopathological problems in children affected by tic disorders – study on a large Italian population. Eur Child Adolesc Psychiatry 13: 166–171

Casey DA, Davis MH (1994) Obsessive-compulsive disorder responsive to electroconvulsive therapy in an elderly woman. South Med J 87: 862–864

Castillo JCR, Castillo ARGL, Biason L, Miguita K, Ikenaga E, Vallada HP (2004) Is 5HT1D-beta involved in the pathogenesis of tic-related OCD? Preliminary results from an OCD paediatric sample ascertained through Tourette's probands. In: Abstracts XIIth World Congress of Psychiatric Genetics. Am J Med Genet Part B: Neuropsychiatr Genet 122B(1): 91

Cath DC, Spinhoven P, Hoogduin CA, Landman AD, van Woerkom TC, van de Wetering BJ, Roos RA, Rooijmans HG (2001a) Repetitive behaviors in Tourette's syndrome and OCD with and without tics: what are the differences? Psychiatry Res 101: 171–185

Cath DC, Spinhoven P, Landman AD, van Kempen GM (2001b) Psychopathology and personality characteristics in relation to blood serotonin in Tourette's syndrome and obsessive-compulsive disorder. J Psychopharmacol 15: 111–119

Cath DC, Spinhoven P, van de Wetering BJ, Hoogduin CA, Landman AD, van Woerkom TC, Roos RA, Rooijmans HG (2000) The relationship between types and severity of repetitive behaviors in Gilles de la Tourette's disorder and obsessive-compulsive disorder. J Clin Psychiatry 61: 505–513

Cavallini MC, Di Bella D, Catalano M, Bellodi L (2000) An association study between 5-HTTLPR polymorphism, COMT polymorphism, and Tourette's syndrome. Psychiatry Res 97: 93–100

Chabane N, Millet B, Delorme R, Lichtermann D, Mathieu F, Laplanche JL, Roy I, Mouren MC, Hankard R, Maier W, Launay JM, Leboyer M (2004) Lack of evidence for association between serotonin transporter gene (5-HTTLPR) and obsessive-compulsive disorder by case control and family association study in humans. Neurosci Lett 363: 154–156

Chae JH, Nahas Z, Wassermann E, Li X, Sethuraman G, Gilbert D, Sallee FR, George MS (2004) A pilot safety study of repetitive transcranial magnetic stimulation (rTMS) in Tourette's syndrome. Cogn Behav Neurol 17: 109–117

Chang HL, Tu MJ, Wang HS (2004) Tourette's syndrome: psychopathology in adolescents. Psychiatr Clin Neurosci 58: 353–358

Chee KY, Sachdev P (1994) The clinical features of Tourette's disorder: an Australian study using a structured interview schedule. Aust NZ J Psychiatry 28: 313–318

Chee KY, Sachdev P (1997) A controlled study of sensory tics in Gilles de la Tourette syndrome and obsessive-compulsive disorder using a structured interview. J Neurol Neurosurg Psychiatry 62: 188–192

Church AJ, Dale RC, Giovannoni G (2004) Anti-basal ganglia antibodies: a possible diagnostic utility in idiopathic movement disorders? Arch Dis Child 89: 611–614

Coffey BJ, Biederman J, Geller DA, Spencer T, Park KS, Shapiro SJ, Garfield SB (2000) The course of Tourette's disorder: a literature review. Harv Rev Psychiatry 8: 192–198

Cohen AJ, Leckman JF (1992) Sensory phenomena associated with Gilles de la Tourette's syndrome. J Clin Psychiatry 53: 319–323

Comer JS, Kendall PC, Franklin ME, Hudson JL, Pimentel SS (2004) Obsessing/worrying about the overlap between obsessive-compulsive disorder and generalized anxiety disorder in youth. Clin Psychol Rev 24: 663–683

Comings DE, Comings BG (1985) Tourette syndrome: clinical and psychological aspects of 250 cases. Am J Hum Genet 37: 435–450

Comings DE, Comings BG (1987) A controlled study of Tourette syndrome. IV. Obsessions, compulsions, and schizoid behaviors. Am J Hum Genet 41: 782–803

Comings DE, Comings BG, Muhleman D, Dietz G, Shahbahrami B, Tast D, Knell E, Kocsis P, Baumgarten R, Kovacs BW, et al. (1991) The dopamine D2 receptor locus as a modifying gene in neuropsychiatric disorders. Jama 266: 1793–1800

Comings DE, Himes JA, Comings BG (1990) An epidemiologic study of Tourette's syndrome in a single school district. J Clin Psychiatry 51: 463–469

Comings DE, MacMurray JP (2003) Maternal age at the birth of the first child as an epistatic factor in psychiatric genetics. In: Abstracts XIth World Congress of Psychiatric Genetics. Am J Med Genet Part B: Neuropsychiatr Genet 122B(1): 52

Comings DE, Rostamkhani M, Emami R, MacMurray JP (2003) Association between the vesicular monoamine transporter VMAT2 and co-morbid symptoms in Tourette's syndrome patients. In: Abstracts XIth World Congress of Psychiatric Genetics. Am J Med Genet Part B: Neuropsychiatr Genet 122B(1): 51

Costello EJ, Angold A, Burns BJ, Stangl DK, Tweed DL, Erkanli A, Worthman CM (1996) The Great Smoky Mountains Study of Youth. Goals, design, methods, and the prevalence of DSM-III-R disorders. Arch Gen Psychiatry 53: 1129–1136

Cruz C, Camarena B, King N, Paez F, Sidenberg D, de la Fuente JR, Nicolini H (1997) Increased prevalence of the seven-repeat variant of the dopamine D4 receptor gene in patients with obsessive-compulsive disorder with tics. Neurosci Lett 231: 1–4

de Groot CM (1997) Course of obsessive-compulsive symptoms in Tourette's syndrome. Depress Anxiety 6: 165–169

de Groot CM, Bornstein RA, Janus MD, Mavissakalian MR (1994) Patterns of obsessive compulsive symptoms in Tourette subjects are independent of severity. Anxiety 1: 268–274

Devor EJ (1984) Complex segregation analysis of Gilles de la Tourette syndrome: further evidence for a major locus mode of transmission. Am J Hum Genet 36: 704–709

Devor EJ, Grandy DK, Civelli O, Litt M, Burgess AK, Isenberg KE, van de Wetering BJ, Oostra B (1990) Genetic linkage is excluded for the D2-dopamine receptor lambda HD2G1 and flanking loci on chromosome 11q22–q23 in Tourette syndrome. Hum Hered 40: 105–108

Diaz-Anzaldua A, Joober R, Riviere JB, Dion Y, Lesperance P, Richer F, Chouinard S, Rouleau GA (2004) Tourette syndrome and dopaminergic genes: a family-based association study in the French Canadian founder population. Mol Psychiatry 9: 272–277

Diniz JB, Rosario-Campos MC, Shavitt RG, Curi M, Hounie AG, Brotto SA, Miguel EC (2004) Impact of age at onset and duration of illness on the expression of comorbidities in obsessive-compulsive disorder. J Clin Psychiatry 65: 22–27

Dougherty DD, Rauch SL, Jenike MA (2004) Pharmacotherapy for obsessive-compulsive disorder. J Clin Psychol 16: 446–455

Drummond LM (1993) The treatment of severe, chronic, resistant obsessive-compulsive disorder. An evaluation of an in-patient programme using behavioural psychotherapy in combination with other treatments. Br J Psychiatry 163: 223–229

Eapen V, Moriarty J, Robertson MM (1994) Stimulus induced behaviours in Tourette's syndrome. J Neurol Neurosurg Psychiatry 57: 853–855

Eapen V, Pauls DL, Robertson MM (1993) Evidence for autosomal dominant transmission in Tourette's syndrome. United Kingdom cohort study. Br J Psychiatry 162: 593–596

Eisenhauer GL, Woody RC (1987) Self-mutilation and Tourette's disorder. J Child Neurol 2: 265–267

Evers RA, van de Wetering BJ (1994) A treatment model for motor tics based on a specific tension-reduction technique. J Behav Ther Exp Psychiatry 25: 255–260

Evidente VG (2000) Is it a tic or Tourette's? Clues for differentiating simple from more complex tic disorders. Postgrad Med 108: 175–176, 179–182

Farid BT (1986) Irritability and resistance in obsessional neurosis. Psychopathology 19: 289–293

Faridi K, Suchowersky O (2003) Gilles de la Tourette's syndrome. Can J Neurol Sci 30 [Suppl 1]: S64–S71

Frankel M, Cummings JL, Robertson MM, Trimble MR, Hill MA, Benson DF (1986) Obsessions and compulsions in Gilles de la Tourette's syndrome. Neurology 36: 378–382

Franklin ME, Kozak MJ, Cashman LA, Coles ME, Rheingold AA, Foa EB (1998) Cognitive-behavioral treatment of pediatric obsessive-compulsive disorder: an open clinical trial. J Am Acad Child Adolesc Psychiatry 37: 412–419

Freeman RD, Fast DK, Burd L, Kerbeshian J, Robertson MM, Sandor P (2000) An international perspective on Tourette syndrome: selected findings from 3,500 individuals in 22 countries. Dev Med Child Neurol 42: 436–447

Gadzicki D, Muller-Vahl KR, Heller D, Ossege S, Nothen MM, Hebebrand J, Stuhrmann M (2004) Tourette syndrome is not caused by mutations in the central cannabinoid receptor (CNR1) gene. Am J Med Genet 127B: 97–103

Gaffney GR, Perry PJ, Lund BC, Bever-Stille KA, Arndt S, Kuperman S (2002) Risperidone versus clonidine in the treatment of children and adolescents with Tourette's syndrome. J Am Acad Child Adolesc Psychiatry 41: 330–336

Gelernter J, Kennedy JL, Grandy DK, Zhou QY, Civelli O, Pauls DL, Pakstis A, Kurlan R, Sunahara RK, Niznik HB, et al. (1993) Exclusion of close linkage of Tourette's syndrome to D1 dopamine receptor. Am J Psychiatry 150: 449–453

Gelernter J, Pakstis AJ, Pauls DL, Kurlan R, Gancher ST, Civelli O, Grandy D, Kidd KK (1990) Gilles de la Tourette syndrome is not linked to D2-dopamine receptor. Arch Gen Psychiatry 47: 1073–1077

Gelernter J, Rao PA, Pauls DL, Hamblin MW, Sibley DR, Kidd KK (1995a) Assignment of the 5HT7 receptor gene (HTR7) to chromosome 10q and exclusion of genetic linkage with Tourette syndrome. Genomics 26: 207–209

Gelernter J, Vandenbergh D, Kruger SD, Pauls DL, Kurlan R, Pakstis AJ, Kidd KK, Uhl G (1995b) The dopamine transporter protein gene (SLC6A3): primary linkage mapping and linkage studies in Tourette syndrome. Genomics 30: 459–463

Geller D, Biederman J, Jones J, Park K, Schwartz S, Shapiro S, Coffey B (1998) Is juvenile obsessive-compulsive disorder a developmental subtype of the disorder? A review of the pediatric literature. J Am Acad Child Adolesc Psychiatry 37: 420–427

Geller DA, Biederman J, Stewart SE, Mullin B, Farrell C, Wagner KD, Emslie G, Carpenter D (2003) Impact of comorbidity on treatment response to paroxetine in pediatric obsessive-compulsive disorder: is the use of exclusion criteria empirically supported in randomized clinical trials? J Child Adolesc Psychopharmacol 13 (Suppl 1): S19–S29

George MS, Trimble MR, Ring HA, Sallee FR, Robertson MM (1993) Obsessions in obsessive-compulsive disorder with and without Gilles de la Tourette's syndrome. Am J Psychiatry 150: 93–97

Giakas WJ (1995) Risperidone treatment for a Tourette's disorder patient with comorbid obsessive-compulsive disorder. Am J Psychiatry 152: 1097–1098

Gilles de la Tourette G (1885) Etude sur une affection nerveuse caracterisee par de l'incoordination motrice accompagnee d'echolalie et de copralalie. Arch Neurol: 19–42, 158–200

Goetz CG, Kompoliti K (2001) Rating scales and quantitative assessment of tics. In: Cohen DJ, Goetz CG, Jankovic J (eds) Tourette syndrome. Lippincott, Williams & Wilkins, New York, pp 31–42

Goetz CG, Tanner CM, Stebbins GT, Leipzig G, Carr WC (1992) Adult tics in Gilles de la Tourette's syndrome: description and risk factors. Neurology 42: 784–788

Grad LR, Pelcovitz D, Olson M, Matthews M, Grad GJ (1987) Obsessive-compulsive symptomatology in children with Tourette's syndrome. J Am Acad Child Adolesc Psychiatry 26: 69–73

Grados MA, Riddle MA, Samuels JF, Liang KY, Hoehn-Saric R, Bienvenu OJ, Walkup JT, Song D, Nestadt G (2001) The familial phenotype of obsessive-compulsive disorder in relation to tic disorders: the Hopkins OCD family study. Biol Psychiatry 50: 559–565

Grados MA, Walkup J, Walford S (2003) Genetics of obsessive-compulsive disorders: new findings and challenges. Brain Dev 25 (Suppl 1): S55–S61

Greenberg BD, Ziemann U, Cora-Locatelli G, Harmon A, Murphy DL, Keel JC, Wassermann EM (2000) Altered cortical excitability in obsessive-compulsive disorder. Neurology 54: 142–147

Grice DE, Leckman JF, Pauls DL, Kurlan R, Kidd KK, Pakstis AJ, Chang FM, Buxbaum JD, Cohen DJ, Gelernter J (1996) Linkage disequilibrium between an allele at the dopamine D4 receptor locus and Tourette syndrome, by the transmission-disequilibrium test. Am J Hum Genet 59: 644–652

Guttmacher LB, Cretella H (1988) Electroconvulsive therapy in one child and three adolescents. J Clin Psychiatry 49: 20–23

Hanna GL, McCracken JT, Cantwell DP (1991) Prolactin in childhood obsessive-compulsive disorder: clinical correlates and response to clomipramine. J Am Acad Child Adolesc Psychiatry 30: 173–178

Hanna PA, Janjua FN, Contant CF, Jankovic J (1999) Bilineal transmission in Tourette syndrome. Neurology 53: 813–818

Hasstedt SJ, Leppert M, Filloux F, van de Wetering BJ, McMahon WM (1995) Intermediate inheritance of Tourette syndrome, assuming assortative mating. Am J Hum Genet 57: 682–689

Hebebrand J, Klug B, Fimmers R, Seuchter SA, Wettke-Schafer R, Deget F, Camps A, Lisch S, Hebebrand K, von Gontard A, Lehmkuhl G, Poustka F, Schmidt M, Baur MP, Remschmidt H (1997) Rates for tic disorders and obsessive compulsive symptomatology in families of children and adolescents with Gilles de la Tourette syndrome. J Psychiatr Res 31: 519–530

Hebebrand J, Nothen MM, Lehmkuhl G, Poustka F, Schmidt M, Propping P, Remschmidt H (1993) Tourette's syndrome and homozygosity for the dopamine D3 receptor gene. German Tourette's Syndrome Collaborative Research Group. Lancet 341: 1483–1484

Hembree EA, Riggs DS, Kozak MJ, Franklin ME, Foa EB (2003) Long-term efficacy of exposure and ritual prevention therapy and serotonergic medications for obsessive-compulsive disorder. CNS Spectr 8: 363–371, 381

Hemmings SMJ, Kinnear CJ, Knowles JA, Lochner C, Moolman-Smook H, Niehaus D, Corfield VA, Stein DJ (2003) Early-versus late-onset obsessive compulsive disorder: clinical and genetic correlates. In: Abstracts XIth World Congress of Psychiatric Genetics. Am J Med Genet Part B: Neuropsychiatr Genet 122B(1): 142

Himle JA, Fischer DJ, Van Etten ML, Janeck AS, Hanna GL (2003) Group behavioral therapy for adolescents with tic-related and non-tic-related obsessive-compulsive disorder. Depress Anxiety 17: 73–77

Hoehn-Saric R, Barksdale VC (1983) Impulsiveness in obsessive-compulsive patients. Br J Psychiatry 143: 177–182

Hoekstra PJ, Anderson GM, Limburg PC, Korf J, Kallenberg CG, Minderaa RB (2004a) Neurobiology and neuroimmunology of Tourette's syndrome: an update. Cell Mol Life Sci 61: 886–898

Hoekstra PJ, Minderaa RB, Kallenberg CG (2004b) Lack of effect of intravenous immunoglobulins on tics: a double-blind placebo-controlled study. J Clin Psychiatry 65: 537–542

Holzer JC, Goodman WK, McDougle CJ, Baer L, Boyarsky BK, Leckman JF, Price LH (1994) Obsessive-compulsive disorder with and without a chronic tic disorder. A comparison of symptoms in 70 patients. Br J Psychiatry 164: 469–473

Hood KK, Baptista-Neto L, Beasley PJ, Lobis R, Pravdova I (2004) Case study: severe self-injurious behavior in comorbid Tourette's disorder and OCD. J Am Acad Child Adolesc Psychiatry 43: 1298–1303

Hoogduin K, Verdellen C, Cath D (1997) Exposure and response prevention in the treatment of Gilles de la Tourette's syndrome: four case studies. Clin Psychol Psychother 4: 125–137

Hornse H, Banerjee S, Zeitlin H, Robertson M (2001) The prevalence of Tourette syndrome in 13-14-year-olds in mainstream schools. J Child Psychol Psychiatry 42: 1035–1039

Hounie AG, Pauls DL, Mercadante MT, Rosario-Campos MC, Shavitt RG, de Mathis MA, de Alvarenga PG, Curi M, Miguel EC (2004) Obsessive-compulsive spectrum disorders in rheumatic fever with and without Sydenham's chorea. J Clin Psychiatry 65: 994–999

Hyde TM, Aaronson BA, Randolph C, Rickler KC, Weinberger DR (1992) Relationship of birth weight to the phenotypic expression of Gilles de la Tourette's syndrome in monozygotic twins. Neurology 42: 652–658

Jankovic J (1997) Tourette syndrome. Phenomenology and classification of tics. Neurol Clin 15: 267–275

Kadesjo B, Gillberg C (2000) Tourette's disorder: epidemiology and comorbidity in primary school children. J Am Acad Child Adolesc Psychiatry 39: 548–555

Karp BI, Hallett M (1996) Extracorporeal 'phantom' tics in Tourette's syndrome. Neurology 46: 38–40

Keck PE Jr, McElroy SL, Strakowski SM, West SA, Sax KW, Hawkins JM, Bourne ML, Haggard P (1998) 12-Month outcome of patients with bipolar disorder following hospitalization for a manic or mixed episode. Am J Psychiatry 155: 646–652

Khalifa N, von Knorring AL (2003) Prevalence of tic disorders and Tourette syndrome in a Swedish school population. Dev Med Child Neurol 45: 315–319

Khanna S, Rajendra PN, Channabasavanna SM (1988) Life events and onset of obsessive compulsive disorder. Int J Soc Psychiatry 34: 305–309

Kim CH, Koo MS, Cheon KA, Ryu YH, Lee JD, Lee HS (2003) Dopamine transporter density of basal ganglia assessed with [123I]IPT SPET in obsessive-compulsive disorder. Eur J Nucl Med Mol Imaging 30: 1637–1643

King RA, Leonard H, March JS (1998) Practice parameters for the assessment and treatment of children and adolescents with obsessive-compulsive disorder. AACAP. J Am Acad Child Adolesc Psychiatry 37: 27S–45S

Kopell BH, Greenberg B, Rezai AR (2004) Deep brain stimulation for psychiatric disorders. J Clin Neurophysiol 21: 51–67

Kuperman S (2002) Tic disorders in the adolescent. Adolesc Med 13: 537–551

Kurlan R (2004) The PANDAS hypothesis: losing its bite? Mov Disord 19: 371–374

Kurlan R, Como PG, Deeley C, McDermott M, McDermott MP (1993) A pilot controlled study of fluoxetine for obsessive-compulsive symptoms in children with Tourette's syndrome. Clin Neuropharmacol 16: 167–172

Kurlan R, Como PG, Miller B, Palumbo D, Deeley C, Andresen EM, Eapen S, McDermott MP (2002) The behavioral spectrum of tic disorders: a community-based study. Neurology 59: 414–420

Kurlan R, Eapen V, Stern J, McDermott MP, Robertson MM (1994) Bilineal transmission in Tourette's syndrome families. Neurology 44: 2336–2342

Kurlan R, Lichter D, Hewitt D (1989) Sensory tics in Tourette's syndrome. Neurology 39: 731–734

Kwak C, Dat Vuong K, Jankovic J (2003) Premonitory sensory phenomenon in Tourette's syndrome. Mov Disord 18: 1530–1533

Lang A (1991) Patient perception of tics and other movement disorders. Neurology 41: 223–228

Lanzi G, Zambrino CA, Termine C, Palestra M, Ferrari Ginevra O, Orcesi S, Manfredi P, Beghi E (2004) Prevalence of tic disorders among primary school students in the city of Pavia, Italy. Arch Dis Child 89: 45–47

Leckman JF (2002) Tourette's syndrome. Lancet 360: 1577–1586

Leckman JF (2003) Phenomenology of tics and natural history of tic disorders. Brain Dev 25 (Suppl 1): S24–S28

Leckman JF, Dolnansky ES, Hardin MT, Clubb M, Walkup JT, Stevenson J, Pauls DL (1990) Perinatal factors in the expression of Tourette's syndrome: an exploratory study. J Am Acad Child Adolesc Psychiatry 29: 220–226

Leckman JF, Grice DE, Barr LC, de Vries AL, Martin C, Cohen DJ, McDougle CJ, Goodman WK, Rasmussen SA (1994a) Tic-related vs. non-tic-related obsessive compulsive disorder. Anxiety 1: 208–215

Leckman JF, King RA, Cohen DJ (1998a) Tics and tic disorders. In: Leckman JF, Cohen DJ (eds) Tourette's syndrome – tics, obsessions, compulsions: developmental psychopathology and clinical care. John Wiley and Sons, New York, pp 23–43

Leckman JF, McDougle CJ, Pauls DL, Peterson BS, Grice DE, King RA, Scahill L, Price LH, Rasmussen SA (2000) Tic-related versus non-tic-related obsessive-compulsive disorder. In: Goodman WK, Rudorfer MV, Maser JD (eds) Obsessive-compulsive disorder: contemporary issues in treatment. Lawrence Erlbaum Associates, Mahwah, pp 43–68

Leckman JF, Peterson BS, Anderson GM, Arnsten AF, Pauls DL, Cohen DJ (1997) Pathogenesis of Tourette's syndrome. J Child Psychol Psychiatry 38: 119–142

Leckman JF, Peterson BS, King RA, Scahill L, Cohen DJ (2001) Phenomenology of tics and natural history of tic disorders. In: Cohen DJ, Goetz CG, Jankovic J (eds) Tourette syndrome. Lippincott, Williams & Wilkins, New York, pp 1–14

Leckman JF, Riddle MA, Hardin MT, Ort SI, Swartz KL, Stevenson J, Cohen DJ (1989) The Yale Global Tic Severity Scale: initial testing of a clinician-rated scale of tic severity. J Am Acad Child Adolesc Psychiatry 28: 566–573

Leckman JF, Walker DE, Cohen DJ (1993) Premonitory urges in Tourette's syndrome. Am J Psychiatry 150: 98–102

Leckman JF, Walker DE, Goodman WK, Pauls DL, Cohen DJ (1994b) 'Just right' perceptions associated with compulsive behavior in Tourette's syndrome. Am J Psychiatry 151: 675–680

Leckman JF, Zhang H, Vitale A, Lahnin F, Lynch K, Bondi C, Kim YS, Peterson BS (1998b) Course of tic severity in Tourette syndrome: the first two decades. Pediatrics 102: 14–19

Lees AJ, Robertson M, Trimble MR, Murray NM (1984) A clinical study of Gilles de la Tourette syndrome in the United Kingdom. J Neurol Neurosurg Psychiatry 47: 1–8

Leonard HL, Lenane MC, Swedo SE, Rettew DC, Gershon ES, Rapoport JL (1992) Tics and Tourette's disorder: a 2- to 7-year follow-up of 54 obsessive-compulsive children. Am J Psychiatry 149: 1244–1251

Lichter DG, Jackson LA, Schachter M (1995) Clinical evidence of genomic imprinting in Tourette's syndrome. Neurology 45: 924–928

Lin H, Yeh CB, Peterson BS, Scahill L, Grantz H, Findley DB, Katsovich L, Otka J, Lombroso PJ, King RA, Leckman JF (2002) Assessment of symptom exacerbations in a longitudinal study of children with Tourette's syndrome or obsessive-compulsive disorder. J Am Acad Child Adolesc Psychiatry 41: 1070–1077

Lombroso PJ, Scahill L, King RA, Lynch KA, Chappell PB, Peterson BS, McDougle CJ, Leckman JF (1995) Risperidone treatment of children and adolescents with chronic tic disorders: a preliminary report. J Am Acad Child Adolesc Psychiatry 34: 1147–1152

Lopez-Ibor JJ Jr (1990) Impulse control in obsessive-compulsive disorder: a biopsychopathological approach. Prog Neuropsychopharmacol Biol Psychiatry 14: 709–718

Luo F, Leckman JF, Katsovich L, Findley D, Grantz H, Tucker DM, Lombroso PJ, King RA, Bessen DE (2004) Prospective longitudinal study of children with tic disorders and/or obsessive-compulsive disorder: relationship of symptom exacerbations to newly acquired streptococcal infections. Pediatrics 113: e578–e585

Maletzky B, McFarland B, Burt A (1994) Refractory obsessive compulsive disorder and ECT. Convuls Ther 10: 34–42

March JS, Franklin M, Nelson A, Foa E (2001) Cognitive-behavioral psychotherapy for pediatric obsessive-compulsive disorder. J Clin Child Psychol 30: 8–18

Marcus D, Kurlan R (2001) Tics and its disorders. Neurol Clin 19: 735–758

Martin JL, Barbanoj MJ, Perez V, Sacristan M (2003) Transcranial magnetic stimulation for the treatment of obsessive-compulsive disorder. Cochrane Database Syst Rev: CD003387

Martino D, Church AJ, Dale RC, Giovannoni G (2004) Antibasal ganglia antibodies and PANDAS. Mov Disord

Mason A, Banerjee S, Eapen V, Zeitlin H, Robertson MM (1998) The prevalence of Tourette syndrome in a mainstream school population. Dev Med Child Neurol 40: 292–296

Mataix-Cols D, Rauch SL, Baer L, Eisen JL, Shera DM, Goodman WK, Rasmussen SA, Jenike MA (2002) Symptom stability in adult obsessive-compulsive disorder: data from a naturalistic two-year follow-up study. Am J Psychiatry 159: 263–268

Mataix-Cols D, Rauch SL, Manzo PA, Jenike MA, Baer L (1999) Use of factor-analyzed symptom dimensions to predict outcome with serotonin reuptake inhibitors and placebo in the treatment of obsessive-compulsive disorder. Am J Psychiatry 156: 1409–1416

Mathews CA, Waller J, Glidden D, Lowe TL, Herrera LD, Budman CL, Erenberg G, Naarden A, Bruun RD, Freimer NB, Reus VI (2004) Self injurious behaviour in Tourette syndrome: correlates with impulsivity and impulse control. J Neurol Neurosurg Psychiatry 75: 1149–1155

McDougle CJ, Goodman WK, Leckman JF, Barr LC, Heninger GR, Price LH (1993) The efficacy of fluvoxamine in obsessive-compulsive disorder: effects of comorbid chronic tic disorder. J Clin Psychopharmacol 13: 354–358

McDougle CJ, Goodman WK, Leckman JF, Lee NC, Heninger GR, Price LH (1994) Haloperidol addition in fluvoxamine-refractory obsessive-compulsive disorder. A double-blind, placebo-controlled study in patients with and without tics. Arch Gen Psychiatry 51: 302–308

Mellman LA, Gorman JM (1984) Successful treatment of obsessive-compulsive disorder with ECT. Am J Psychiatry 141: 596–597

Miguel EC, Baer L, Coffey BJ, Rauch SL, Savage CR, O'sullivan RL, Phillips K, Moretti C, Leckman JF, Jenike MA (1997) Phenomenological differences appearing with repetitive behaviours in obsessive-compulsive disorder and Gilles de la Tourette's syndrome. Br J Psychiatry 170: 140–145

Miguel EC, do Rosario-Campos MC, Prado HS, do Valle R, Rauch SL, Coffey BJ, Baer L, Savage CR, O'sullivan RL, Jenike MA, Leckman JF (2000) Sensory phenomena in obsessive-compulsive disorder and Tourette's disorder. J Clin Psychiatry 61: 150–156; quiz 157

Miguel EC, do Rosario-Campos MC, Shavitt RG, Hounie AG, Mercadante MT (2001) The tic-related obsessive-compulsive disorder phenotype and treatment implications. Adv Neurol 85: 43–55

Miguel EC, Shavitt RG, Ferrao YA, Brotto SA, Diniz JB (2003) How to treat OCD in patients with Tourette syndrome. J Psychosom Res 55: 49–57

Millet B, Chabane N, Delorme R, Leboyer M, Leroy S, Poirier MF, Bourdel MC, Mouren-Simeoni MC, Rouillon F, Loo H, Krebs MO (2003) Association between the dopamine receptor D4 (DRD4) gene and obsessive-compulsive disorder. Am J Med Genet 116B: 55–59

Mink JW (2001) Neurobiology of basal ganglia circuits in Tourette syndrome: faulty inhibition of unwanted motor patterns? Adv Neurol 85: 113–122

Moll GH, Eysenbach K, Woerner W, Banaschewski T, Schmidt MH, Rothenberger A (2000) Quantitative and qualitative aspects of obsessive-compulsive behaviour in children with attention-deficit hyperactivity disorder compared with tic disorder. Acta Psychiatr Scand 101: 389–394

Moll GH, Rothenberger A (1999) [Relationship between tics and compulsion]. Nervenarzt 70: 1–10

Moriarty J, Eapen V, Costa DC, Gacinovic S, Trimble M, Ell PJ, Robertson MM (1997) HMPAO SPET does not distinguish obsessive-compulsive and tic syndromes in families multiply affected with Gilles de la Tourette's syndrome. Psychol Med 27: 737–740

Müller SV, Johannes S, Wieringa B, Weber A, Muller-Vahl K, Matzke M, Kolbe H, Dengler R, Munte TF (2003) Disturbed monitoring and response inhibition in patients with Gilles de la Tourette syndrome and co-morbid obsessive compulsive disorder. Behav Neurol 14: 29–37

Murphy ML, Pichichero ME (2002) Prospective identification and treatment of children with pediatric autoimmune neuropsychiatric disorder associated with group A streptococcal infection (PANDAS). Arch Pediatr Adolesc Med 156: 356–361

Murphy TK, Sajid M, Soto O, Shapira N, Edge P, Yang M, Lewis MH, Goodman WK (2004) Detecting pediatric autoimmune neuropsychiatric disorders associated with streptococcus in children with obsessive-compulsive disorder and tics. Biol Psychiatry 55: 61–68

Nee LE, Caine ED, Polinsky RJ, Eldridge R, Ebert MH (1980) Gilles de la Tourette syndrome: clinical and family study of 50 cases. Ann Neurol 7: 41–49

Nestadt G, Addington A, Samuels J, Liang KY, Bienvenu OJ, Riddle M, Grados M, Hoehn-Saric R, Cullen B (2003) The identification of OCD-related subgroups based on comorbidity. Biol Psychiatry 53: 914–920

Nestadt G, Samuels J, Riddle M, Bienvenu OJ 3rd, Liang KY, LaBuda M, Walkup J, Grados M, Hoehn-Saric R (2000) A family study of obsessive-compulsive disorder. Arch Gen Psychiatry 57: 358–363

Neziroglu F, Anemone R, Yaryura-Tobias JA (1992) Onset of obsessive-compulsive disorder in pregnancy. Am J Psychiatry 149: 947–950

Nicolini H, Cruz C, Paez F, Camarena B (1998) [Dopamine D2 and D4 receptor genes distinguish the clinical presence of tics in obsessive-compulsive disorder]. Gac Med Mex 134: 521–527

Nomoto F, Machiyama Y (1990) An epidemiological study of tics. Jpn J Psychiatry Neurol 44: 649–655

Nordstrom EJ, Burton FH (2002) A transgenic model of comorbid Tourette's syndrome and obsessive-compulsive disorder circuitry. Mol Psychiatry 7: 617–625, 524

O'Connor KP (2001) Clinical and psychological features distinguishing obsessive-compulsive and chronic tic disorders. Clin Psychol Rev 21: 631–660

Palumbo D, Maughan A, Kurlan R (1997) Hypothesis III. Tourette syndrome is only one of several causes of a developmental basal ganglia syndrome. Arch Neurol 54: 475–483

Pappert EJ, Goetz CG, Louis ED, Blasucci L, Leurgans S (2003) Objective assessments of longitudinal outcome in Gilles de la Tourette's syndrome. Neurology 61: 936–940

Pauls DL (2003) An update on the genetics of Gilles de la Tourette syndrome. J Psychosom Res 55: 7–12

Pauls DL, Alsobrook JP, Almasy L, Leckman JF, Cohen DJ (1991a) Genetic and epidemiological analyses of the Yale Tourette's Syndrome Family Study data. Psychiatr Genet 2: 28

Pauls DL, Alsobrook JP 2nd, Goodman W, Rasmussen S, Leckman JF (1995) A family study of obsessive-compulsive disorder. Am J Psychiatry 152: 76–84

Pauls DL, Leckman JF (1986) The inheritance of Gilles de la Tourette's syndrome and associated behaviors. Evidence for autosomal dominant transmission. N Engl J Med 315: 993–997

Pauls DL, Raymond CL, Stevenson JM, Leckman JF (1991b) A family study of Gilles de la Tourette syndrome. Am J Hum Genet 48: 154–163

Perugi G, Akiskal HS, Gemignani A, Pfanner C, Presta S, Milanfranchi A, Lensi P, Ravagli S, Maremmani I, Cassano GB (1998) Episodic course in obsessive-compulsive disorder. Eur Arch Psychiatry Clin Neurosci 248: 240–244

Peterson BS (2001c) Neuroimaging studies of Tourette syndrome: a decade of progress. Adv Neurol 85: 179–196

Peterson BS, Leckman JF (1998) The temporal dynamics of tics in Gilles de la Tourette syndrome. Biol Psychiatry 44: 1337–1348

Peterson BS, Pine DS, Cohen P, Brook JS (2001a) Prospective, longitudinal study of tic, obsessive-compulsive, and attention-deficit/hyperactivity disorders in an epidemiological sample. J Am Acad Child Adolesc Psychiatry 40: 685–695

Peterson BS, Staib L, Scahill L, Zhang H, Anderson C, Leckman JF, Cohen DJ, Gore JC, Albert J, Webster R (2001b) Regional brain and ventricular volumes in Tourette syndrome. Arch Gen Psychiatry 58: 427–440

Peterson BS, Thomas P, Kane MJ, Scahill L, Zhang H, Bronen R, King RA, Leckman JF, Staib L (2003) Basal ganglia volumes in patients with Gilles de la Tourette syndrome. Arch Gen Psychiatry 60: 415–424

Piacentini J, Bergman RL, Jacobs C, McCracken JT, Kretchman J (2002) Open trial of cognitive behavior therapy for childhood obsessive-compulsive disorder. J Anxiety Disord 16: 207–219

Price RA, Kidd KK, Cohen DJ, Pauls DL, Leckman JF (1985) A twin study of Tourette syndrome. Arch Gen Psychiatry 42: 815–820

Rapoport M, Feder V, Sandor P (1998) Response of major depression and Tourette's syndrome to ECT: a case report. Psychosom Med 60: 528–529

Rauch SL, Whalen PJ, Curran T, Shin LM, Coffey BJ, Savage CR, McInerney SC, Baer L, Jenike MA (2001) Probing striato-thalamic function in obsessive-compulsive disorder and Tourette syndrome using neuroimaging methods. Adv Neurol 85: 207–224

Ravizza L, Barzega G, Bellino S, Bogetto F, Maina G (1995) Predictors of drug treatment response in obsessive-compulsive disorder. J Clin Psychiatry 56: 368–373

Ravizza L, Maina G, Bogetto F (1997) Episodic and chronic obsessive-compulsive disorder. Depress Anxiety 6: 154–158

Ravizza L, Maina G, Torta RFB (1991) Are serotonergic antidepressants more effective in episodic' obsessive-compulsive disorder? In: Cassano GB, Akiskal HS (eds) Serotonin-related psychiatric syndromes: clinical and therapeutic links. Royal Society of Medicine Services, London, pp 61–65

Robertson MM (1989) The Gilles de la Tourette syndrome: the current status. Br J Psychiatry 154: 147–169

Robertson MM (1994) Annotation: Gilles de la Tourette syndrome-an update. J Child Psychol Psychiatry 35: 597–611

Robertson MM (2000) Tourette syndrome, associated conditions and the complexities of treatment. Brain 123 Pt 3: 425–462

Robertson MM, Banerjee S, Kurlan R, Cohen DJ, Leckman JF, McMahon W, Pauls DL, Sandor P, van de Wetering BJ (1999) The Tourette syndrome diagnostic confidence index: development and clinical associations. Neurology 53: 2108–2112

Robertson MM, Gourdie A (1990) Familial Tourette's syndrome in a large British pedigree. Associated psychopathology, severity, and potential for linkage analysis. Br J Psychiatry 156: 515–521

Robertson MM, Trimble MR, Lees AJ (1988) The psychopathology of the Gilles de la Tourette syndrome. A phenomenological analysis. Br J Psychiatry 152: 383–390

Robertson MM, Trimble MR, Lees AJ (1989) Self-injurious behaviour and the Gilles de la Tourette syndrome: a clinical study and review of the literature. Psychol Med 19: 611–625

Roessner V, Banaschewski T, Rothenberger A (2004) Therapy of tic-disorders. Z Kinder Jugendpsychiatr Psychother 32: 245–263

Rosario-Campos MC, Leckman JF, Mercadante MT, Shavitt RG, Prado HS, Sada P, Zamignani D, Miguel EC (2001) Adults with early-onset obsessive-compulsive disorder. Am J Psychiatry 158: 1899–1903

Rosenberg LA, Brown J, Singer HS (1995) Behavioral problems and severity of tics. J Clin Psychol 51: 760–767

Rothenberger A, Banaschewski T (2004) Tic-disorders. In: Grillberg C, Harrington R, Steinhausen HC (eds) A clinican's handbook of child and adolsecent psychiatry. Cambridge University Press, Cambridge

Rothenberger A, Banaschewski T, Roessner V (2005) Tic-Störungen. In: Herpetz-Dahlmann B, Resch F, Schulte-Markwort M, Warnke A (eds) Entwicklungspsychiatrie. Schattauer, Stuttgart

Saba PR, Dastur K, Keshavan MS, Katerji MA (1998) Obsessive-compulsive disorder, Tourette's syndrome, and basal ganglia pathology on MRI. J Neuropsychiatr Clin Neurosci 10: 116–117

Sachdev PS, McBride R, Loo CK, Mitchell PB, Malhi GS, Croker VM (2001) Right versus left prefrontal transcranial magnetic stimulation for obsessive-compulsive disorder: a preliminary investigation. J Clin Psychiatry 62: 981–984

Santangelo SL, Pauls DL, Goldstein JM, Faraone SV, Tsuang MT, Leckman JF (1994) Tourette's syndrome: what are the influences of gender and comorbid obsessive-compulsive disorder? J Am Acad Child Adolesc Psychiatry 33: 795–804

Saxena S, Rauch SL (2000) Functional neuroimaging and the neuroanatomy of obsessive-compulsive disorder. Psychiatr Clin North Am 23: 563–586

Scahill L, Chappell PB, King RA, Leckman JF (2000) Pharmacologic treatment of tic disorders. Child Adolesc Psychiatr Clin North Am 9: 99–117

Scahill L, Riddle MA, King RA, Hardin MT, Rasmusson A, Makuch RW, Leckman JF (1997) Fluoxetine has no marked effect on tic symptoms in patients with Tourette's syndrome: a double-blind placebo-controlled study. J Child Adolesc Psychopharmacol 7: 75–85

Scahill L, Tanner C, Dure L (2001) The epidemiology of tics and Tourette syndrome in children and adolescents. Adv Neurol 85: 261–271

Scahill LD, Leckman JF, Marek KL (1995) Sensory phenomena in Tourette's syndrome. Adv Neurol 65: 273–280

Schoenian S, Konig I, Oertel W, Remschmidt H, Ziegler A, Hebebrand J, Bandmann O (2003) HLA-DRB genotyping in Gilles de la Tourette patients and their parents. Am J Med Genet 119B: 60–64

Seuchter SA, Hebebrand J, Klug B, Knapp M, Lehmkuhl G, Poustka F, Schmidt M, Remschmidt H, Baur MP (2000) Complex segregation analysis of families ascertained through Gilles de la Tourette syndrome. Genet Epidemiol 18: 33–47

Shapiro AK, Shapiro ES, Young JG, Feinberg TE (1988) Gilles de la Tourette Syndrome. Raven Press, New York

Silva RR, Munoz DM, Barickman J, Friedhoff AJ (1995) Environmental factors and related fluctuation of symptoms in children and adolescents with Tourette's disorder. J Child Psychol Psychiatry 36: 305–312

Singer HS, Giuliano JD, Zimmerman AM, Walkup JT (2000) Infection: a stimulus for tic disorders. Pediatr Neurol 22: 380–383

Singer HS, Loiselle CR, Lee O, Minzer K, Swedo S, Grus FH (2004) Anti-basal ganglia antibodies in PANDAS. Mov Disord 19: 406–415

Singer HS, Walkup JT (1991) Tourette syndrome and other tic disorders. Diagnosis, pathophysiology, and treatment. Medicine (Baltimore) 70: 15–32

Snider LA, Swedo SE (2003) Childhood-onset obsessive-compulsive disorder and tic disorders: case report and literature review. J Child Adolesc Psychopharmacol 13 (Suppl 1): S81–S88

Stefl ME (1984) Mental health needs associated with Tourette syndrome. Am J Publ Health 74: 1310–1313

Stein DJ, Hollander E, Simeon D, Cohen L (1994) Impulsivity scores in patients with obsessive-compulsive disorder. J Nerv Ment Dis 182: 240–241

Steketee G, Eisen J, Dyck I, Warshaw M, Rasmussen S (1999) Predictors of course in obsessive-compulsive disorder. Psychiatry Res 89: 229–238

Stephens RJ, Bassel C, Sandor P (2004) Olanzapine in the treatment of aggression and tics in children with Tourette's syndrome – a pilot study. J Child Adolesc Psychopharmacol 14: 255–266

Stephens RJ, Sandor P (1999) Aggressive behaviour in children with Tourette syndrome and comorbid attention-deficit hyperactivity disorder and obsessive-compulsive disorder. Can J Psychiatry 44: 1036–1042

Stewart SE, Geller DA, Jenike M, Pauls D, Shaw D, Mullin B, Faraone SV (2004) Long-term outcome of pediatric obsessive-compulsive disorder: a meta-analysis and qualitative review of the literature. Acta Psychiatr Scand 110: 4–13

Stober G, Hebebrand J, Cichon S, Bruss M, Bonisch H, Lehmkuhl G, Poustka F, Schmidt M, Remschmidt H, Propping P, Nothen MM (1999) Tourette syndrome and the norepinephrine transporter gene: results of a systematic mutation screening. Am J Med Genet 88: 158–163

Stokes A, Bawden HN, Camfield PR, Backman JE, Dooley JM (1991) Peer problems in Tourette's disorder. Pediatrics 87: 936–942

Strassnig M, Riedel M, Muller N (2004) Electroconvulsive therapy in a patient with Tourette's syndrome and co-morbid obsessive compulsive disorder. World J Biol Psychiatry 5: 164–166

Sukhodolsky DG, Scahill L, Zhang H, Peterson BS, King RA, Lombroso PJ, Katsovich L, Findley D, Leckman JF (2003) Disruptive behavior in children with Tourette's syndrome: association with ADHD comorbidity, tic severity, and functional impairment. J Am Acad Child Adolesc Psychiatry 42: 98–105

Swedo SE, Leonard HL, Garvey M, Mittleman B, Allen AJ, Perlmutter S, Lougee L, Dow S, Zamkoff J, Dubbert BK (1998) Pediatric autoimmune neuropsychiatric disorders associated with streptococcal infections: clinical description of the first 50 cases. Am J Psychiatry 155: 264–271

Swerdlow NR (2001) Obsessive-compulsive disorder and tic syndromes. Med Clin North Am 85: 735–755

Swerdlow NR, Gierz M, Berkowitz A, Nemiroff R, Lohr J (1990) Electroconvulsive therapy in a patient with severe tic disorder and major depressive episode. J Clin Psychiatry 51: 34–35

Swerdlow NR, Zinner S, Farber RH, Seacrist C, Hartston HJ (1999) Symptoms in obsessive-compulsive disorder and Tourette syndrome: a spectrum? CNS Spectrums 4: 21–33

Tass PA, Klosterkotter J, Schneider F, Lenartz D, Koulousakis A, Sturm V (2003) Obsessive-compulsive disorder: development of demand-controlled deep brain stimulation with methods from stochastic phase resetting. Neuropsychopharmacology 28 (Suppl 1): S27–S34

Tekin S, Cummings JL (2002) Frontal-subcortical neuronal circuits and clinical neuropsychiatry: an update. J Psychosom Res 53: 647–654

Thomas SG, Kellner CH (2003) Remission of major depression and obsessive-compulsive disorder after a single unilateral ECT. J Ect 19: 50–51

Tolin DF, Abramowitz JS, Przeworski A, Foa EB (2002) Thought suppression in obsessive-compulsive disorder. Behav Res Ther 40: 1255–1274

Tolin DF, Maltby N, Diefenbach GJ, Hannan SE, Worhunsky P (2004) Cognitive-behavioral therapy for medication nonresponders with obsessive-compulsive disorder: a wait-list-controlled open trial. J Clin Psychiatry 65: 922–931

Trivedi HK, Mendelowitz AJ, Fink M (2003) Gilles de la Tourette form of catatonia: response to ECT. J Ect 19: 115–117

Turpin G (1983) The behavioural management of tic disorders: a critical review. Adv Behav Res Ther 5: 203–245

Urraca N, Camarena B, Gomez-Caudillo L, Esmer MC, Nicolini H (2004) Mu opioid receptor gene as a candidate for the study of obsessive compulsive disorder with and without tics. Am J Med Genet 127B: 94–96

Vandenbergh DJ, Thompson MD, Cook EH, Bendahhou E, Nguyen T, Krasowski MD, Zarrabian D, Comings D, Sellers EM, Tyndale RF, George SR, O'Dowd BF, Uhl GR (2000) Human dopamine transporter gene: coding region conservation among normal, Tourette's disorder, alcohol dependence and attention-deficit hyperactivity disorder populations. Mol Psychiatry 5: 283–292

Van Noppen B, Steketee G, McCorkle BH, Pato M (1997) Group and multifamily behavioral treatment for obsessive compulsive disorder: a pilot study. J Anxiety Disord 11: 431–446

Verdellen CW, Keijsers GP, Cath DC, Hoogduin CA (2004) Exposure with response prevention versus habit reversal in Tourettes's syndrome: a controlled study. Behav Res Ther 42: 501–511

Verhulst FC, van der Ende J, Ferdinand RF, Kasius MC (1997) The prevalence of DSM-III-R diagnoses in a national sample of Dutch adolescents. Arch Gen Psychiatry 54: 329–336

Visser-Vandewalle V, Temel Y, van der Linden Ch, Ackermans L, Beuls E (2004) Deep brain stimulation in movement disorders. The applications reconsidered. Acta Neurol Belg 104: 33–36

Walkup JT, LaBuda MC, Singer HS, Brown J, Riddle MA, Hurko O (1996) Family study and segregation analysis of Tourette syndrome: evidence for a mixed model of inheritance. Am J Hum Genet 59: 684–693

Walkup JT, Rosenberg LA, Brown J, Singer HS (1992) The validity of instruments measuring tic severity in Tourette's syndrome. J Am Acad Child Adolesc Psychiatry 31: 472–477

Wang HS, Kuo MF (2003) Tourette's syndrome in Taiwan: an epidemiological study of tic disorders in an elementary school at Taipei County. Brain Dev 25 (Suppl 1): S29–S31

Wilhelm S, Deckersbach T, Coffey BJ, Bohne A, Peterson AL, Baer L (2003) Habit reversal versus supportive psychotherapy for Tourette's disorder: a randomized controlled trial. Am J Psychiatry 160: 1175–1177

Woods DW, Twohig MP, Flessner CA, Roloff TJ (2003) Treatment of vocal tics in children with Tourette syndrome: investigating the efficacy of habit reversal. J Appl Behav Anal 36: 109–112

Xu C, Ozbay F, Wigg K, Shulman R, Tahir E, Yazgan Y, Sandor P, Barr CL (2003) Evaluation of the genes for the adrenergic receptors alpha 2A and alpha 1C and Gilles de la Tourette Syndrome. Am J Med Genet 119B: 54–59

Yaryura-Tobias JA, Rabinowitz DC, Neziroglu F (2003) Possible basal ganglia pathology in children with complex symptoms. J Clin Psychiatry 64: 1495–1501

Zhang H, Leckman JF, Pauls DL, Tsai CP, Kidd KK, Campos MR (2002) Genomewide scan of hoarding in sib pairs in which both sibs have Gilles de la Tourette syndrome. Am J Hum Genet 70: 896–904

Ziemann U, Paulus W, Rothenberger A (1997) Decreased motor inhibition in Tourette's disorder: evidence from transcranial magnetic stimulation. Am J Psychiatry 154: 1277–1284

Zohar AH, Pauls DL, Ratzoni G, Apter A, Dycian A, Binder M, King R, Leckman JF, Kron S, Cohen DJ (1997) Obsessive-compulsive disorder with and without tics in an epidemiological sample of adolescents. Am J Psychiatry 154: 274–276

Zohar AH, Ratzoni G, Pauls DL, Apter A, Bleich A, Kron S, Rappaport M, Weizman A, Cohen DJ (1992) An epidemiological study of obsessive-compulsive disorder and related disorders in Israeli adolescents. J Am Acad Child Adolesc Psychiatry 31: 1057–1061

Authors' address: Dr. V. Roessner, Department of Child and Adolescent Psychiatry, University of Göttingen, Von-Siebold-Strasse 5, 37075 Göttingen, Germany, e-mail: vroessn@gwdg.de

The effectiveness of interventions for children with autism[*]

P. Howlin

Department of Community Health Sciences, St. George's Hospital Medical School,
Tooting, London, United Kingdom

Summary. Over the past 50 years very many different treatments have been promoted as bringing about significant improvements, or even cures, for children with autism. However, few interventions involve controlled studies of any kind; randomised control trials are virtually non-existent and when appropriate research methodology has been applied the results are generally far from positive. Recent research suggests that the most effective results stem from early intensive behavioural interventions. Although many questions remain concerning the optimal age at which treatment should begin, the intensity of treatment and the many other variables that may affect outcome, there is growing evidence of *general* strategies that can be effective in ameliorating the problems associated with autism.

Introduction

In the earliest accounts of autism the condition was generally viewed as a psychiatric disorder with a psychogenic basis (Szurek and Berlin, 1956; Kanner, 1951) and many psychiatrists like Kanner assumed it to be a form of childhood schizophrenia. Consequently, psychoanalysis, together with the drugs and other treatments used for patients with schizophrenia (including ECT) were widely used (see Campbell, 1978). However, in the mid to late 1960's, autism began to be viewed as a behavioural disorder, with many studies demonstrating the effectiveness of operant approaches (Bandura, 1969; Ullman and Krasner, 1965). The focus was generally on the elimination of "undesirable" behaviours, notably tantrums, aggression or self injury, with frequent use of aversive procedures, including electric shock (see Howlin and Rutter, 1987) and treatment was largely conducted on an inpatient, hospital basis with very little involvement of the child's family in therapy. The procedures used to increase skills such as social interactions or communication were often highly prescriptive and inflexible, and took little note of individual factors such as the child's developmental level, or the family situation.

During the 1970's, largely due to the influential work of Michael Rutter (1972), recognition of the fundamental cognitive, social and communication

---

[*] The general content of this paper is based on a chapter on interventions for autism in Howlin P (2004) Autism and Asperger Syndrome: preparing for adulthood. Routledge, London

deficits underlying the disorder led to a shift to more individually based treatment programmes; home based interventions began to replace inpatient hospital treatment and there was much wider use of naturalistic teaching and reinforcement strategies. This trend continued throughout the 1980's with increasing integration of home and school based programmes, greater involvement of typically developing peers in therapy and a steady movement towards more inclusive education. There was growing recognition, too, of the need for early intervention and of the role played by communication deficits in causing many of the "challenging behaviours" frequently associated with autism. Reactions against abuses arising from the uncontrolled use of aversive procedures led to a focus on the development of more positive treatment strategies. It was in the 1980's, too, that Lorna Wing (1981) highlighted the needs of children with autism who were of normal intellectual ability and had relatively well developed language skill, in other words children with Asperger syndrome (Asperger, 1944).

In the last decade, therapeutic work in the field of autism has been characterized by a number of both positive and less positive trends. On the positive side there have been many attempts to extend functional analytic approaches to intervention. Recognition that communication deficits are frequently at the root of many problem behaviours (Durand and Merges, 2001; Greenspan and Wieder, 1999) has also had a major influence on therapeutic practice. There has been an increased focus on developmentally based approaches and much greater awareness of the importance of enhancing generalized communication skills in young children with autism (Prizant et al., 1997). Naturalistic approaches to intervention have replaced the more prescriptive behavioural programmes, with greater reliance on naturally occurring environmental reinforcers, and recognition of the need to encourage self initiation and self motivation (Prizant and Rubin, 1999). "Pivotal" response training and social skills programmes have also helped to improve social and communicative interactions (Bauminger, 2002; Koegel and Koegel, 1995; Koegel et al., 1999). There have even been attempts to improve the fundamental deficits associated with autism, such as impairments in "Theory of Mind" (Baron Cohen, 2002; Howlin et al., 1998).

Pharmacological interventions

Despite the growth of individually based approaches to the treatment of autism, there is still widespread use of medications to control behavioural disturbance, even for very young children (Gringras, 2000; McDougle, 1997). Among the many different pharmacological agents that have been used are the "one size fits all" type (such as fenfluramine) that have been claimed to have a positive impact on almost all aspects of children's functioning. Then there are more specific agents including SSRI's (fluoxitine, fluvoxamine); other anti-depressants, such as clomipramine; stimulants (mainly methylphenidate); anti-hypertensive agents (clonidine); anti-psychotics (haloperidol); opioid antagonists (naltrexone) to treat self injurious behaviour; mood stabilizers, such as lithium, and anti-convulsants. Many other agents have also been recommended, including melatonin, megavitamins, even the use of a 36 ingredient vitamin/mineral/anti-oxidant supplement, and procedures to reduce mercury levels in the body (c.f. Rimland, 2000).

The use of psychotropic medication for young children with autism varies greatly from country to country. In the UK there is relatively little use of pharmacological treatments for autism per se. although, of course, medication may be necessary for comorbid conditions such as epilepsy (Gringras, 2000). This is not the case in the US (Posey and McDougle, 2001) where pharmaceutical companies even promote drugs for toddlers with autism. Despite the high rates of prescribing in countries such as the US, there are few randomized control trials of the use of psychotropic medications in autism and little information about long-term effects, especially when given to young children. For example, fenfluramine, which during the 1970's to 80's was widely used for children with autism in the US, has now been largely withdrawn because of concerns about serious side effects and potential long-term damage (see Campbell et al., 1996). Another recent treatment, extensively publicised by the media, involves injections with secretin (a gastro-intestinal peptide hormone). This has been claimed to have almost "miraculous" effects (Horvath et al., 1998; Rimland, 1998), with rapid improvements in behaviour and language being cited. However, a recent comprehensive review, involving around 600 children (Esch and Carr, 2004) found that 12 out of 13 placebo-controlled studies failed to demonstrate any positive effects.

Dietary and vitamin treatments for autism have also increased in popularity and are widely recommended in numerous Internet websites. The cleverly named "Eye Q" supplement, for example is currently receiving considerable publicity in the UK. However, as is the case with so many interventions publicised on the Internet, there is almost no controlled experimental evaluation of these treatments. The Autism Network for Dietary Intervention (www.autismndi.com) recently listed nearly 100 studies relating to food allergy and autism, claiming that there is "significant scientific evidence to support a trial period of careful elimination of these proteins for the diet of children on the autistic spectrum". However, many of the studies listed are not, in fact, directly related to autism, and there is a dearth of double blind trials – which are the only sure way of establishing whether intervention is actually successful. A recent Cochrane review of 18 studies of vitamin B6 and Magnesium treatments for autism (Nye and Brice, 2003) found that only one (Findling et al., 1997) involved randomized, double-blind allocation to treatment or control conditions. This study showed no benefit of magnesium and B6 compared to placebo. Another Cochrane review of gluten and casein free diets for children with autism (Millward et al., 2004) found only one small scale study that met basic research criteria, and this reported only limited effects.

Educational programmes

The importance of structured educational programmes has been recognised for many years, since research by Rutter and Bartak (1973) confirmed that autistic children exposed to structured, task oriented, "academic" programmes made significantly better educational and social progress than children in less structured environments. The TEACCH programme (Schopler and Mesibov, 1995; Schopler, 1997) provides a framework for teaching that emphasises the need for structure, appropriate environmental organisation and the use of clear visual cues to circumvent communication difficulties. The programme also takes account of developmental levels and the importance of individually based teaching, as well as incorporating behavioural and cognitive approaches. A recent controlled study by Ozonoff and Cathcart (1998) reported significant short-term gains in pre-school children with autism following the introduction of a daily TEACCH session into their daily home programme. Another, small scale study, comparing 8 children with autism and severe intellectual disability enrolled in a TEACCH programme with 8 in an integrated schooling programme, found that, although children in both groups made progress over 12 months, improvements in the TEACCH group were greater (Panieri et al., 2002).

A number of other, mostly US based models exist. Among the best evaluated of these are the Denver model (Rogers et al., 1987); the Douglass centre programme (Harris et al., 1995); the Individualized Support Programme (Dunlap and Fox, 1999) and the LEAP programme (Strain and Hoyson, 2000) (see National Research Council, 2001 for review). In the UK the National Autistic Society promotes the SPELL (Structure, Positive, Empathy, Low Arousal, Links) approach. Other programmes focus on the encouragement of play and pleasurable interactions between pre-school children with autism and their parents or peers. These include the Developmental Intervention Model (Greenspan and Wieder, 1999); the Waldon Program (McGee et al., 1987), the Hanen approach (Sussman, 1999) and the Early Bird Project (Shields, 2001). However, there have been no large scale, independent evaluations of these interventions. There is also an increasing number of programmes specifically designed to overcome social-communication impairments in young children with autism. The "Bright Start Programme" (Butera and Haywood, 1995) focuses on the development of cognitive and meta-cognitive abilities. Koegel and Koegel (1995) illustrate how traditional behavioural techniques can be successfully adapted for use in more naturalistic school settings. The potential value of computer based teaching has also been demonstrated in a number of small scale projects (Bernard-Opitz et al., 1999; Bosseler and Massaro, 2003; Moore and Calvert, 2000; Tjus et al., 2001).

Two approaches that have become widely incorporated into teaching programmes for children with autism over the last few years are the Picture Exchange Communication System (PECS; Bondy and Frost, 1996) in which children are taught to use symbols and pictures to enhance communication skills, and Social Stories (Gray, 1995) which employs cartoon-type illustrations to help children understand how to respond in social situations. Again, although there are many anecdotal or single case accounts of the value of these two approaches (many written by the proponents themselves) independent, controlled studies are lacking. A recent review of Social Stories concluded that, although the underlying rationale is strong, there is little research evidence to demonstrate their effectiveness (Sansosti et al., 2004). Similarly, independent evaluations of PECS (Charlop-Christy et al., 2002; Magiati and Howlin, 2003;

Kravits et al., 2002; Schwarz et al., 1998; Tincani, 2004), whilst reporting some positive gains in children's non-verbal communication, found fewer improvements in their spoken language skills.

Early, behaviourally based intervention programmes

In recent years there has been a steady growth in early intervention programmes for toddlers and pre-school children with autism. These are designed to help parents and teachers develop appropriately structured and consistent management strategies during the child's early years, which, in principle, should enhance developmental progress and minimise later behavioural problems (see Rogers, 1996). A variety of developmental, educational and behavioural approaches has been found to have positive effects, with significant improvements being reported in language and social behaviours, self care, motor and academic skills (Dawson and Osterling, 1997; Rogers, 1998). When control groups have been involved (which is by no means always the case) the gains made by the experimental children have generally been greater, with more children in the treatment groups subsequently being accepted into mainstream school. Nevertheless, although children's overall level of functioning appears to be enhanced by programmes of this kind, there is less evidence of a marked reduction in autistic symptomatology. This conclusion holds even for the very early, intensive behavioural interventions (EIBI) of Lovaas and his colleagues (Lovaas, 1996). These have been reported as bringing about major changes in children's cognitive ability (sometimes as much as 30 IQ points or more), and it is claimed that around 40% of the children involved become "indistinguishable" from their normally developing peers. However, such claims have been disputed and it is evident that the way in which IQ is measured, both prior to and following intervention, can have a significant impact on results (Magiati and Howlin, 2001). The restricted range of the outcome measures used in these early interventions studies has also been criticised (Gresham and MacMillan, 1998). Moreover, recent re-analysis of the data published by Lovaas and his colleagues suggests that the claim that 47% of children attain normal functioning is not substantiated. Instead, in most EIBI programmes, although children clearly show improvements, none appear to have "recovered" from their autism (Shea, 2004).

Generally, the number of cases involved in evaluative studies of early behavioural/educational interventions remains very small, and blind, randomised control trials are virtually non-existent (Lord, 2000). Many other questions remain to be answered concerning the *specific* effects of these early programmes, since the content is often very eclectic and the relative importance of the different components of treatment is unknown. There are also questions about the comparative merits of one-to-one vs. group teaching, or home-based vs. school-based programmes. Similarly, surprisingly little is known about the characteristics of the children who appear to respond best to programmes of this kind. Thus, although several studies indicate that IQ and language levels are important predictive variables (Harris and Handleman, 2000), with the most able children generally making most progress, this is not invariably the case (Koegel, 2000). The optimal length of time in therapy is another issue. Lovaas

(1996) has proposed that 40 hours a week of therapy, over two years or more is required, although positive results have been reported for less intensive behavioural programmes (Gabriels and Hill, 2001). On the whole, the more successful early intervention programmes appear to involve a minimum of around 15 to 20 hours a week, last at least 6 months, and require a relatively high adult child ratio (Rogers, 1996). The active participation of parents in therapy is also important (Schreibman, 2000). Finally, but perhaps most importantly, longer-term evaluations, covering many different aspects of functioning are required in order to evaluate the true effectiveness and cost benefits of these early, and often very costly, programmes.

"Alternative" interventions for autism

Autism has probably attracted more attention within the field of "alternative medicine" than almost any other developmental disorder and claims for miracle treatments and "cures" abound. On offer are numerous dietary and vitamin treatments; endocrine and other injections; physical therapies (including intensive and systematic exercise, "Facilitated Communication", Holding Therapy, cranial osteopathy, and swimming with dolphins); sensory therapies (scotopic sensitivity training; sensory integration; auditory integration, and music therapy) and "psycho-educational" therapies, such as the Waldon or Son-Rise programmes (for review see Howlin, 2004). Listed below, in alphabetical order, are just some of the approaches that have received widespread (if sometimes short lived) media publicity over recent years.

Auditory Integration Training (AIT)

This involves listening to electronically processed music through headphones for a total of 10 hours, (usually in 2×30 minute sessions over a 10 day period). The training device uses filters to dampen peak frequencies to which the participants are said to be "hypersensitive". AIT is claimed to result in a dramatic reduction in autistic symptomatology (c.f. "The Sound of a Miracle: A Child's Triumph over Autism"; Stehli, 1992) and was widely promoted in Australia, Europe and the US during the late 1980's/early 90's (Rimland and Edelson, 1994, 1995).

Cranial osteopathy

This involves very gentle manipulation of various parts of the body, particularly the head. It is claimed that a disturbed pattern of motion in the frontal lobes of the brain can sometimes be identified, or that the whole head is tight and unyielding. Treatment may last for several months, and the effects are said to range from minor reductions in hyperactivity to major improvements in communication (NAS 1997).

Daily Life Therapy and the Higashi schools

"Daily Life Therapy", as practised in the Japanese run Higashi schools has been claimed to produce unprecedented progress in children with autism (Kitahara,

1983, 1984a, b). The focus of the curriculum is on group activities, with a vigorous physical education programme, much music, art and drama. The high anxiety levels of many children with autism are said to be reduced by physical exercise, which releases the endorphins controlling anxiety and frustration. There is rigorous control of challenging and inappropriate behaviours, but individuality is not encouraged and there is relatively little emphasis on the development of spontaneous communication skills.

Facilitated Communication

A facilitator supports the client's hand, wrist or arm whilst he or she uses a keyboard, or letter board, to spell out words, phrases or sentences. The use of facilitated communication with people with autism is based on the theory that many of their difficulties result from a physical inability to express themselves, rather than more fundamental social or communication deficits. The facilitator should presume that the client possesses unrecognised literacy skills and the provision of physical support can then lead to "Communication Unbound" (Biklen, 1990).

Floor Time

Includes child directed "interactive experiences", in a low stimulus environment, for two to five hours a day. Greenspan (1998) stipulates that "the therapeutic program must begin as soon as possible so that the children and their parents are re-engaged in emotional interactions that use their emerging, but not yet fully developing capacities for communication.... The longer such children remain uncommunicative...the more deeply the children tend to withdraw and become perseverative and self-stimulatory". Floor time helps to "transform this perseveration into interaction". Once this occurs, the child will begin to show more purposeful behaviour to imitate gestures, sounds and play. It is claimed that children enrolled in the programme between the ages of 18 and 30 months subsequently become "fully communicative (using complex sentences adaptively), creative, warm, loving, and joyful" (Greenspan, 1998).

Gentle Teaching

"Gentle Teaching" is defined as "a non-aversive method of reducing challenging behaviour that aims to teach bonding and interdependence through gentleness, respect and solidarity". Emphasis is placed on "the importance of unconditional valuing in the caregiving and therapeutic process" (Jones and McCaughy, 1992). The approach was claimed to be successful for all individuals with learning difficulties and challenging behaviours (McGee, 1985) and rose to popularity in the wake of growing concerns about the use of aversive procedures in the treatment of people with autism or other learning disabilities.

Holding therapy

"Holding" was initially promoted in the U.S. by Martha Welch (1988), who claimed it was effective for a wide range of problems, from autism to marital difficulties. It was also publicised widely in Germany (Prekop, 1984), Italy (Zappella, 1988) and the U.K. (Richer and Zappella, 1989). Therapy involves holding the child tightly until he or she accepts comfort. Central to this is the requirement to provoke a state of distress, in order that the child will need to be comforted. Richer and Zappella (1989) claimed that this approach "had a major contribution to make to the treatment of autistic children" and that it could result in their becoming "entirely normal".

Movement therapies

Conductive education which involves "patterning" or systematic-exercising of autistic children by their parents, and usually teams of volunteers, has also been advocated as a potential cure for autism (Delacato, 1974; Cummins, 1988). The stimulation of muscle activity in a controlled way, often throughout many hours of the day, is claimed to repair damaged or non-functional neural networks. Vigorous exercise has been reported in a number of studies to have a positive effect on behavioural problems and is a crucial component in Daily Life Therapy (see above) There are also suggestions that it may play a role in the effectiveness of holding therapy (Welch, 1988). Parents have reported various behavioural improvements following physical exercise (Rimland, 1988), and reductions in stereotyped, disruptive and hyperactive behaviours, sleep disturbance, aggression, anxiety, self injury, and depression have been noted in other studies. Vigorous exercise has also been claimed to improve attention span, social skills, work performance and cognitive functioning, and to reduce self-stimulatory behaviours in individuals with autism, as well as other forms of learning disability (see Elliott et al., 1994; Rosenthall-Malek and Mitchell, 1997).

Music therapy

Although mostly used as one component of a broader educational programme for children with autism, there are claims that music therapy alone can play "a significant role in developing...emotional, integrative and self organisational experiences" (Trevarthen et al., 1998). However, the term covers a wide variety of different techniques, and reports of its effectiveness often incorporate additional interventions, such as psychoanalysis or play therapy.

Pet therapies

Claims of apparently dramatic improvements in behaviour after exposure to pet therapy of various kinds make occasional appearances in the media, and the positive effects of swimming with dolphins have received particular publicity. However, there is now a growing movement in California to protect dolphins from being used for the benefits of human beings, and the specific or long-term benefits of these approaches have never been assessed.

Psychoanalytic psychotherapy

Kanner's comments (1943) on the lack of warmth shown by parents of children with autism and their tendency towards a "mechanization of human contacts" led many to view the condition as being predominantly psychogenic in origin. It was variously suggested that autism was due to a lack of stimulation, parental rejection, lack of warmth, or deviant family interactions (Bettleheim, 1967; Boatman and Szurek, 1960; O'Gorman, 1970). Such theories had a profound and widespread influence on therapeutic practice, and for many years individual psychotherapy (mainly in the form of psychoanalytically oriented non-directive play therapy) was considered the treatment of choice (Szurek and Berlin, 1956; Goldfarb, 1961). Although Campbell et al. (1996), in a general view of interventions concluded that psychoanalysis is of "limited value" the approach is still viewed as beneficial by some (e.g. Hobson, 2002).

The Son Rise Programme (formerly the Option method)

This approach is based on the premise that the child with autism finds the world confusing and distressing and hence attempts to shut it out. This then starves the brain of the stimuli needed to develop social interaction skills, thereby further increasing confusion and reinforcing the desire for isolation. The essential principle is to make social interactions pleasurable, and to ensure that involvement with *people* becomes more attractive than involvement in obsessional or ritualistic behaviours. Problem behaviours should be viewed as an understandable reaction to children's difficulties in making sense of or controlling their world (Kaufman, 1977, 1981). In order to "reach" the child with autism, adults must be prepared to join in with and enjoy the activities that the child finds pleasurable (very often his or her obsessional activities). Parents are taught to become more aware of the cues given by their own children and to respond more effectively to these. After 9,000 hours of such treatment the Kaufmans' own son is said to have progressed from being "a severely autistic child...with an IQ of about 30" to a completely normal young man with "a near genius IQ" (c.f. A Miracle to Believe In, 1981).

Scotopic sensitivity training

Scotopic sensitivity, or sensitivity to certain wave lengths of light is said to result in a many different symptoms, including reading and communication difficulties, spatial and perceptual deficits, and attentional problems. Special spectacles, incorporating lenses of a variety of different colours, can be designed to provide the "optimum" tint for each individual and are reported to bring about improvements in body and spatial awareness, eye contact, communication and self control in many different disorders, including autism (Irlen, 1995). Donna Williams, is claimed to have found the results "close to miraculous...she was able to listen and concentrate better; her speech became more fluent and spontaneous".

Sensory integration therapy

Many children with autism have problems in dealing with complex sensory stimuli (Minshew et al., 1997). Sensory integration therapy aims to improve sensory processing and increase sensory awareness and responsivity by using a variety of stimuli, such as swings, balls, trampolines, soft brushes and cloths for rubbing the skin, perfume, massage, coloured lights or objects with unusual textures (Ayres, 1979). "Deep pressure therapy" (rolling children up tightly in mats or mattresses), may also be involved. Rimland (1995) reported that around a quarter of programmes for autistic children in the U.S. were utilising this approach.

Interpreting treatment claims

Unfortunately, despite the impressive claims, few of these methods have been subject to any form of experimental investigation; there are no randomised comparison trials or even well controlled single case or small group studies. Instead, information on outcome tends to be based on a few, mostly anecdotal single case reports; there is no information on long term effectiveness, and publicity is rarely afforded to families for whom the treatments did not work. Facilitated Communication (FC), Auditory Integration Training (AIT) and Sensory-Integration programmes are amongst the very few therapies that have been subject to experimental evaluation. Because of its widespread use in the US, and an increasing number of legal cases in which false accusations of (mostly sexual) abuse were made during facilitated sessions, Facilitated Communication has now been the focus of at least 50 studies involving several hundred subjects (see reviews by Green, 1994; Jacobsen et al., 1995; Mostert, 2001; Simpson and Myles, 1993). These have clearly demonstrated that there is virtually no evidence of independent communication. Instead all the evidence points to the fact that the communications are directed by the facilitator, not the client with autism. Moreover, so extensive have been the concerns over abuses arising from the use of this technique that, in 1994, the American Psychological Association adopted the resolution that: "Facilitated Communication is a controversial and unproved procedure with no scientifically demonstrated support for its efficacy". Similarly, the American Academy of Pediatrics Committee on Children with Disabilities (1998) concluded that "there are good scientific data showing (FC) to be ineffective. Moreover. . .the potential for harm does exist, particularly if unsubstantiated accusations of abuse occur using FC". However, although the method is now widely discredited among researchers, its occasional use within schools continues (The Times, Court Report, July 13, 2000).

There are also a few evaluative studies of Auditory Integration Therapy (see Dawson and Watling, 2000 for general review), although most of these have involved very small numbers of subjects. A recent Cochrane review of Auditory Integration Training and other auditory therapies (Sinha et al., 2004) concluded that the data in most of these studies were "unusable" and the 3 studies that met basic experimental criteria showed no effect of therapy. In general there is no evidence that AIT produces any greater benefits than placebo or control conditions and the American Academy of Pediatrics Committee (1998) concluded, "there are no good controlled studies to support its use". This committee also recommended that the use of either Facilitated Communication or Auditory Integration Training "does not appear warranted at this time, except within research protocols".

Table 1. Research adequacy (New York Health Dept. review)

Therapy	Total articles	% Meeting criteria
Behavioural/education interventions	300	8%
Other interventions (FC; Auditory Integration etc.)	63	5%
Drugs	99	12%
Vitamins, diet etc.	44	7%

Sensory-integration procedures have been the focus of much more limited research, despite their widespread use within many educational settings. In a recent review, Dawson and Watling (2000) were able to identify only 4 evaluative studies, involving 26 children in total. Although some positive outcomes were reported, the fact that no study involved a comparison group meant that no conclusions could be drawn concerning effectiveness.

In recent years there have been several comprehensive reviews of the effectiveness of interventions for young children with autism The New York Health State Department Review (1999) of interventions for pre-school children with autism highlighted the poor quality of much of the research in this area and, as is apparent from Table 1, of the hundreds of published papers reviewed, only a minority met basic criteria for experimental research. This report concluded that there was no evidence for the effectiveness of many therapies, including sensory integration, touch therapy or auditory integration. The use of Facilitated Communication was "strongly discouraged". Of the various medical or dietary interventions reviewed (Secretin, immunoglobulin injections, anti-yeast treatments, vitamin or dietary manipulations) again there was little, if any, evidence of effectiveness, and on the whole, because of serious concerns about side-effects or long-term sequelae, these were not recommended. There was more evidence in favour of pharmacological treatments, but little information on the likely benefits and disadvantages for specific sub groups of children and serious concerns were raised about the long-term effects, particularly when used with very young children. A report from the Maine Autism Task Force (2000) also concluded that there was no peer reviewed, scientific evaluation for treatments such as Floor time (Greenspan, 1998), and the Son Rise Program (Kaufman, 1997) was found to be "without scientific evaluation of any kind". The existing evidence for the effectiveness of auditory integration, sensory integration or TEACCH was deemed "inadequate". Facilitated Communication was considered to be potentially harmful and lacking in evidence. The report also emphasises that is the duty of professionals to disclose information on the current inadequacy of evidence for these interventions "to key decision makers influencing the child's intervention".

Generally similar conclusions concerning treatment effectiveness were reached by the UK "National Autism Plan for Children" (le Couteur et al., 2003). The most positive findings, in each of these reviews, related to behavioural and educational programmes. However, both the UK and New York reports concluded that although applied behavioural analysis techniques *in general* have a positive outcome, there was no evidence in favour of any one specific approach. It appeared that interventions of moderate intensity (i.e. around 20 hours a week) produced better results than shorter programmes, but there was no evidence that programmes of 40 hours or more a week provided greater benefits. The involvement of parents in therapy was viewed as important, and programmes with a focus on reducing behavioural problems, improving communication, or enhancing social interaction showed positive outcomes. These findings are generally endorsed by other research in this area. Thus, Sheinkopf and Siegel (1998) concluded that early behavioural/educational interventions are a good option for children with autism, and certainly far better than no intervention or non-specialist school placements. However, they found no evidence in favour of any one approach, any one level of intensity, or any particular degree of structure. Similarly, Prizant and Rubin (1999) note that, given the current state of research in the field, no one approach has been demonstrated to be superior to all others, or to be equally effective for all children.

Evidence in support of the value of early intervention?

It is widely accepted that early intervention is vital in helping children with autism to develop essential skills in the earliest years, and in preventing the escalation of later behavioural difficulties. The claims, particularly by Lovaas and his colleagues, that intervention is most effective if it can begin between the ages of 2 to 4 years has led to a push towards earlier and earlier educational and behavioural programmes. Indeed, in order to ensure access to pre-school intervention, much research over the last decade has concentrated on improving facilities and techniques to ensure early identification and diagnosis (Lord, 1995). However, surprisingly, there is almost no empirical evidence to support the assertion that early intervention results in more favourable long-term outcomes. Several studies do report positive outcomes for children enrolled in intervention programmes prior to 4 years of age (Anderson et al., 1987; Birnbrauer and Leach, 1993; Sheinkopf and Siegel, 1998) but these have not conducted systematic comparisons between children of different ages. Lovaas (1993) noted that the younger children in his intervention studies did much better than those who were older, but again there was no direct comparison between children who began therapy at the recommended age, (i.e. around 2) and those who started later, at around 4 or 5 years. Fenske et al. (1985) conducted a small scale, comparative study of 18 children, 9 aged under 5 years, and 9 aged over 5 when therapy began. More children in the early treatment group went on to mainstream school than in the intervention group. However, school placement was the only outcome measure utilised and, crucially, the 2 groups were not matched prior to the onset of treatment. Recent findings by Stone and Yoder (2001), in showing that the amount of time in language therapy from the age of 2 tends to predict outcome at 4, might also be cited in support of the argument that "earlier = better". Similarly, Harris and Handleman (2000) found that children admitted to a specialist pre-school programme before the age of $3\frac{1}{2}$ were more likely subsequently to be placed in a regular educational classroom than those who were aged on average $4\frac{1}{2}$ when pre-school intervention began. However, outcome, in terms of later educational placement was also significantly related to pre-school IQ measures, and the relative importance of IQ vs. age was not explored.

Rogers (1998) notes that "the hypothesis that age at start of treatment is an important variable in determining outcome has tremendous implications for the field and needs to be tested with methodologically rigorous designs". Unfortunately, no such designs have yet been employed. Certainly, in the absence of any evidence to the contrary, it would seem to make common sense (and in reality that is all we have to go on) to ensure that families of young children with autism are offered appropriate help as soon as possible after diagnosis. Given the rigid behaviour patterns of children with autism, it is clear that once problem behaviours are established, it can be very difficult to change these. Thus, the earlier effective management strategies can be put into place, and appropriate patterns of behaviour established, the less are the chances of problem behaviours developing in the future. It is also evident that certain behaviours, whilst entirely acceptable in very young children, become increasingly less so as individuals grow older. Informed advice to parents, concerning the types of behaviour that may lead to potential problems with age can also have important preventative effects (Howlin, 1998). There is a danger, however, that a single-minded focus on the importance of early, pre-school intervention could have a negative impact on older children with autism. Despite improvements in the age of diagnosis over recent years, many children, particularly those who are more able, do not receive a definitive diagnosis until they reach junior school, or even later (Howlin and Asgharian, 1999). For them, or for the thousands of children who for a variety of other reasons have no access to early intervention, an assumption of "better late than never" is more appropriate than "early intervention or nothing". Harris and Handleman (2000), for example, noted that even the older children in their study made important progress and they are explicit that their data should "not be taken to suggest that children 4 years of age and older should be denied intensive treatment". Whatever the age at which an individual's problems are recognised, appropriate strategies can and should be put into place to help deal with these and there is considerable research indicating that many individuals with autism continue to make considerable improvements as they grow older (Gilchrist et al., 2001; Howlin, 2003; Howlin et al., 2004; Mawhood Howlin and Rutter, 2000; Mesibov et al., 1989; Piven et al., 1996; Seltzer et al., 2003). Indeed, for some, particularly those who are more able, adolescence can often be a period of remarkable improvement and change (Kanner, 1973). This is an age at which some children, at least, become more aware of their difficulties and of how they can moderate their behaviours in order to improve social interactions. Unfortunately, there are very few intervention programmes geared specifically for the needs of this age group, and this may mean that both they, their families, and the professionals involved in their care are missing out on a crucial opportunity for change.

Conclusions

It is clear, given the current state of research in the field of autism, that no single approach has been demonstrated to be superior to all others or to be equally effective for all individuals. Indeed, given the complexity of autism and the range of difficulties and skills shown by these children, expectations that a single therapy will succeed with everyone are clearly unrealistic. Prizant and Rubin (1999) note that the knowledge base for intervention programmes should derive from a combination of different sources, including theory (developmental, learning, family systems etc), clinical and educational data, knowledge about best practice, and empirical data from well designed small group and single case studies. Such information can then be used to indicate *components* of treatment that are likely to be beneficial but these components must then be adapted to the needs of each individual and his or her family. The following guidelines may help to improve daily life for many families:

— Treatment programmes should be individually designed to take account of the individual's cognitive level, the severity of autistic symptomatology and overall developmental level. (Koegel et al., 2001). Chronological age and general temperament/personality are also important factors to consider.
— Structured educational/daily living programmes, with an emphasis on visually based cues can provide the individual with autism with a predictable and readily understandable environment, thereby minimizing confusion and distress (Schopler, 1997)
— Interventions should take account of the core deficits of autism. Much can be achieved by ensuring that the communication used by others is appropriate for the individual's *comprehension* level and that verbal messages are augmented by visual cues. Programmes with a focus on social-communication deficits associated with autism may also have significant effects (see Rogers, 2000). Stereotyped and ritualistic tendencies frequently become progressively more unacceptable with age and thus should be effectively managed from early childhood (Howlin, 2004).
— Many so-called undesirable or challenging behaviours are a reflection of limited behavioural repertoires or poor communication skills. A focus on skill enhancement, and the establishment of more effective communication strategies is often the most successful means of reducing difficult or disruptive behaviours (Durand and Merges, 2001).
— Treatment approaches that are family centred result in greater generalisation and maintenance of skills. The development of management strategies that can be implemented consistently but in ways that do not demand extensive sacrifice in terms of time, money or other aspects of family life, seems most likely to offer benefits for all involved (Marcus et al., 1997). Practical support from skilled professionals can be crucial for families in the early years. Professional advice should also help families to make contact with appropriate parent organisations, educational and social services networks, and to find assistance, if necessary, with the financial burden that raising a child with a disability so often entails.

References

American Academy of Pediatrics (1998) Auditory integration training and facilitated communication for autism. Pediatrics 102: 431–433
American Psychological Association (1994) Resolution on facilitated communication. August 1994

Anderson SR, Avery DL, DiPietro EK, Edwards GL, Christian WP (1987) Intensive home-based early intervention with autistic children. Educ Treat Child 10: 352–366

Asperger H (1944) Autistic psychopathy in childhood (translated and annotated by editor). In: Frith U (ed) (1991) Autism and Asperger Syndrome. Cambridge University Press, Cambridge

Autism Network for Dietary Intervention (www.autismndi.com)

Ayres JA (1979) Sensory integration and the child. Western Psychology Service, Los Angeles

Bandura A (1969) Principles of behavior modification. Holt, Rinehart and Winston, New York

Baron-Cohen S (2002) Mind reading – the interactive guide to emotions. User guide and resource pack. University of Cambridge, Cambridge

Bauminger N (2002) The facilitation of social-emotional understanding and social interaction in high-functioning children with autism: intervention outcomes. J Autism Dev Disord 32: 283–298

Bernard-Opitz V, Sriram N, Sapuan S (1999) Enhancing vocal limitations in children with autism using the IBM SpeechViewer. Autism: Int J Res Pract 3: 131–147

Bettleheim B (1967) The empty fortress: infantile autism and the birth of the self. Free Press, New York

Biklen D (1990) Communication unbound: autism and praxis. Harvard Educ Rev 60: 291–315

Birnbrauer JS, Leach DJ (1993) The Murdoch early intervention program after 2 years. Behav Change 10: 63–74

Boatman M, Szurek S (1960) A clinical study of childhood schizophrenia. In: Jackson D (ed) The etiology of schizophrenia. Basic Books, New York

Bondy A, Frost L (1996) Educational approaches in pre-school: behavior techniques in a public school setting. In: Schopler E, Mesibov GB (eds) Learning and cognition in autism. Plenum Press, New York, pp 311–334

Bosseler A, Massaro DW (2003) Development and evaluation of a computer-animated tutor for vocabulary and language learning in children with autism. J Autism Dev Disord 33: 653–672

Butera G, Haywood HC (1995) Cognitive education of young children with autism: an application of Bright Start. In: Schopler E, Mesibov G (eds) Learning and cognition in autism. Plenum Press, New York

Campbell M (1978) Pharmacotherapy. In: Rutter M, Schopler E (eds) Autism: a reappraisal of concepts and treatment. Plenum Press, New York, pp 337–355

Campbell M, Schopler E, Cueva JE, Hallin A (1996) Treatment of autistic disorder. J Am Acad Child Adolesc Psychiatry 35: 134–143

Charlop-Christy MH, Carpenter M, LeBlanc LA, Kellett K (2002) Using the Picture Exchange Communication System (PECS) with children with autism: assessment of PECS acquisition speech social-communicative behavior and problem behavior. J Appl Behav Analy 35: 213–231

Cummins RA (1988) The neurologically impaired child: Doman-Delacato techniques reappraisal. Croom Helm, London

Dawson G, Osterling J (1997) Early intervention in autism. In: Guralnick M (ed) The effectiveness of early intervention. Brookes Publishing Co, Baltimore, pp 307–326

Dawson G, Watling R (2000) Interventions to facilitate auditory visual and motor integration in autism: a review of the evidence. J Autism Dev Disord 30: 415–422

Delacato CH (1974) The ultimate stranger: the autistic child. Doubleday, New York

Dunlap G, Fox L (1999) A demonstration of behavioral support for young children with autism. J Positive Behav Intervent 1: 77–87

Durand VM, Merges E (2001) Functional communication training: a contemporary behavior analytic intervention for problem behavior. Focus Autism Dev Disord 16: 110–119

Elliott RO, Dobbin AR, Rose GD, Soper HV (1994) Vigorous aerobic exercise versus general motor training: effects on maladaptive and stereotypic behavior of adults with autism and mental retardation. J Autism Dev Disord 25: 565–576

Esch BE, Carr JE (2004) Secretin as a treatment for autism: a review of the evidence. J Autism Dev Disord 34: 543–555

Fenske EC, Zalenki S, Krantz PJ, McClannahan LE (1985) Age at intervention and treatment outcome for autistic children in a comprehensive intervention program. Anal Intervent Dev Disabil 5: 49–58

Findling RL, Maxwell K, Scotese-Wojtila L, Husang J, Yamashita T, Wiznitzer M (1997) High-dose pyridoxine and magnesium administration in children with autistic disorder: An absence of salutary effects in a double-blind placebo-controlled study. J Autism Dev Disabil 27: 467–478

Gabriels RL, Hill DE (2001) Autism – from research to individualized practice. Jessica Kingsley Publishers, London and Philadelphia

Gilchrist A, Green J, Cox A, Rutter M, Le Couteur A (2001) Development and current functioning in adolescents with Asperger Syndrome: a comparative study. J Child Psychol Psychiatry 42: 227–240

Goldfarb W (1961) Growth and change of schizophrenic children. Wiley, New York

Green G (1994) The quality of the evidence. In: Shane HC (ed) Facilitated communication: the clinical and social phenomenon. Singular Press, San Diego, pp 157–226

Greenspan SI (1998) A developmental approach to problems in relating and communicating in autistic spectrum disorders and related syndromes. Spotlight Topics Dev Disabil 1: 1–6

Greenspan SJ, Wieder S (1999) A functional developmental approach to autism spectrum disorders. J Assoc Persons Severe Handicap 3: 147–161

Gresham FM, Macmillan DL (1998) Early Intervention Project: can its claims be substantiated and replicated. J Autism Dev Disord 28: 5–13

Gray CA (1995) Teaching children with autism to 'read' social situations In: Quill KA (ed) Teaching children with autism: strategies to enhance communication and socialization. Delmar, New York, pp 219–242

Gringras P (2000) Practical paediatric psychopharmacological prescribing in autism: the potential and the pitfalls. Autism: Int J Res Pract 4: 229–243

Harris SL, Handleman JS (2000) Age and IQ at intake as predictors of placement for young children with autism: a four- to six-year follow-up. J Autism Dev Disord 30: 137–141

Harris SL, Handleman JS, Belchic J, Glasberg B (1995) The Vineland Adaptive Behavior Scales for young children with autism. Spec Services Schools 10: 45–52

Hobson P (2002) The cradle of thought. Macmillan, London

Horvath K, Stefanalos G, Sokolski KN, Wachtel R, Nabors L, Tildon JT (1998) Improved social and language skills after secretin administration in patients with autistic spectrum disorders. J Assoc Acad Minority Phys 9: 9–15

Howlin P (1998) Children with Autism and Asperger Syndrome: guide for practitioners and carers. Wiley, London

Howlin P (2003) Outcome in high-functioning adults with autism with and without early language delays: implications for the differentiation between autism and Asperger syndrome. J Autism Dev Disord 33: 3–13

Howlin P (2004) Autism and Asperger syndrome: preparing for adulthood, 2nd ed. Routledge, London

Howlin P, Asgharian A (1999) The diagnosis of autism and Asperger syndrome: findings from a survey of 770 families. Dev Med Child Neurol 41: 834–839

Howlin P, Rutter M (1987) The consequences of language delay for other aspects of development. In: Yule W, Rutter M (eds) Language development and disorders. Mac Keith Press, Oxford, pp 271–294

Howlin P, Baron-Cohen S, Hadwin J, Swettenham J (1998) Teaching children with autism to mindread. A practical manual for parents and teachers. Wiley, Chichester

Howlin P, Goode S, Hutton J, Rutter M (2004) Adult outcome for children with autism. J Child Psychol Psychiatry 45: 212–229

Irlen H (1995) Viewing the world through rose tinted glasses. Communication 29: 8–9

Jacobson JW, Mulick JA, Schwartz AA (1995) A history of facilitated communication: science pseudoscience and anti-science. Am Psychol 50: 750–765

Jones RSP, McCaughey RE (1992) Gentle teaching and applied behavior analysis. A critical review. J Appl Behav Anal 25: 853–867

Kanner J (1951) The conception of wholes and parts in early infantile autism. Am J Psychiatry 108: 23–26

Kanner L (1943) Autistic disturbances of affective contact. Nerv Child 2: 217–250

Kanner L (1973) Childhood psychosis: initial studies and new insights. Winston/Wiley, New York

Kaufman BN (1977) To love is to be happy with. Fawcett Crest, New York

Kaufman BN (1981) A miracle to believe in. Doubleday, New York

Kaufman BN (1997) Son rise: the miracle continues. Option Indigo Press, Sheffield MA

Kitahara K (1983) Daily life therapy, vol 1. Musashino Higashi Gakuen School, Tokyo

Kitahara K (1984a, b) Daily life therapy, vol 2, 3. Musashino Higashi Gakuen, Tokyo

Koegel LK (2000) Interventions to facilitate communication in autism. J Autism Dev Disord 30: 383–392

Koegel RL, Koegel LK (1995) Teaching children with autism: strategies for initiating positive interactions and improving learning opportunities. Brookes, Baltimore

Koegel LK, Koegel RL, Harrower JK, Carter CM (1999) Pivotal response intervention. I. Overview of approach. J Assoc Persons Severe Handicaps 24: 174–185

Koegel RL, Koegel LK, McNerney EK (2001) Pivotal areas in intervention for autism. J Clin Child Psychol 30: 19–32

Kravits TE, Kamps DM, Kemmerer K, Potucek J (2002) Brief report: increasing communication skills for an elementary-aged student with autism using the picture exchange communication system. J Autism Dev Disord 32: 225–230

Le Couteur A (2003) National Autism Plan for Children (NAPC). Produced by NIASA National Initiative for Autism Screening and Assessment. National Autistic Society, London

Lord C (1995) Facilitating social inclusion: examples from peer intervention programs. In: Schopler E, Mesibov G (eds) Learning and cognition in autism. Plenum Press, New York, pp 221–239

Lord C (2000) Commentary: Achievements and future directions for intervention research in communication and autism spectrum disorders. J Autism Dev Disord 306: 393–398

Lovaas OI (1993) The development of a treatment – research project for developmentally disabled and autistic children. J Appl Behav Anal 26: 617–630

Lovaas OI (1996) The UCLA young autism model of service delivery. In: Maurice C (ed) Behavioral intervention for young children with autism. Pro-Ed, Austin, pp 241–250

Magiati I, Howlin P (2001) Monitoring the progress of preschool children with autism enrolled in early intervention programmes. Autism: Int J Res Pract 5: 399–406

Magiati I, Howlin P (2003) A pilot evaluation study of the Picture Exchange Communication System (PECS) for children with autistic spectrum disorders. Autism: Int J Res Pract 7: 297–320

Maine Administrators of Services for Children with Disabilities (MADSEC) (2000) Autism Task Force Report

Marcus LM, Kunce LJ, Schopler E (1997) Working with families. In: Cohen D, Volkmar F (eds) Handbook of autism and pervasive developmental disorders, 2nd edn. Wiley, New York, pp 631–649

Mawhood L, Howlin P, Rutter M (2000) Autism and developmental receptive language disorder – a follow-up comparison in early adult life. I. Cognitive and language outcomes. J Child Psychol Psychiatry 41: 547–559

McDougle CJ (1997) Psychopharmacology. In: Cohen DJ, Volkmar FR (eds) Handbook of autism and pervasive developmental disorders, 2nd edn. John Wiley, New York, pp 707–729

McGee JJ (1985) Gentle teaching. Mental Handicap in New Zealand 9: 13–24

McGee JJ, Menolascino PE, Hobbs DC, Menousek PE (1987) Gentle teaching: a non-aversive approach to helping persons with mental retardation. Human Science Press, New York

Mesibov GB, Schopler E, Schaffer B, Michal N (1989) Use of the Childhood Autism Rating Scale with autistic adolescents and adults. J Am Acad Child Adolesc Psychiatry 28: 538–541

Millward C, Ferriter M, Calver S, Connell-Jones G (2004) Gluten- and casein-free diets for autistic spectrum disorder (Cochrane Review). The Cochrane Library Issue 4. John Wiley & Sons, Chichester

Minshew NJ, Sweeney JA, Bauman ML (1997) Neurological aspects of autism. In: Cohen DJ, Volkmar FR (eds) Handbook of autism and pervasive developmental disorders, 2nd edn. John Wiley, New York, pp 344–369

Moore M, Calvert S (2000) Brief report: Vocabulary acquisition for children with autism: teacher or computer instruction. J Autism Dev Disord 30: 359–362

Mostert MP (2001) Facilitated communication since 1995: a review of published studies. J Autism Dev Disord 31: 287–313

National Autistic Society (1997) Approaches to autism. National Autistic Society, London

National Research Council (2001) Educating children with autism. Committee on Educational Interventions for Children with Autism, Division of Behavioral and Social Sciences and Education National Research Council. National Academy Press, Washington DC

New York Health State Department (1999) Clinical practice guidelines for assessment and intervention for young children (age 0–3 years) with autism/pervasive developmental disorder. Early Intervention Program, New York State Department of Health

Nye C, Brice A (2003) Combined vitamin B6-magnesium treatment in autism spectrum disorder. Cochrane Database of Systematic Reviews 4 CD003497

O'Gorman G (1970) The nature of childhood autism, 2nd edn. Butterworth, London

Ozonoff S, Cathcart K (1998) Effectiveness of a home program intervention for young children with autism. J Autism Dev Disord 28: 25–32

Panerai S, Ferrante L, Zingale M (2002) Benefits of the Treatment and Education of Autistic and Communication Handicapped Children (TEACCH) programme as compared with a non-specific approach. J Intellect Disabil Res 46: 318–327

Piven J, Harper J, Palmer P, Arndt S (1996) Course of behavioral change in autism: a retrospective study of high-IQ adolescents and adults. J Am Acad Child Psychiatry 35: 523–529

Posey DJ, McDougle CJ (2001) The pharmacotherapy of target symptoms associated with autistic disorder and other pervasive developmental disorders. Harvard Rev Psychiatry 8: 45–63

Prekop JL (1984) Zur Festhalte Therapie bei Autistischen Kindern. Der Kinderarzt 15: 798–802

Prizant BM, Rubin E (1999) Contemporary issues in interventions for autism spectrum disorders: a commentary. J Assoc Persons with Severe Handicaps 24: 199–208

Prizant B, Schuler A, Wetherby A, Rydell P (1997) Enhancing language and communication development: language approaches. In: Cohen D, Volkmar F (eds) Handbook of autism and pervasive developmental disorders, 2nd edn. Wiley, New York, pp 572–605

Richer J, Zappella M (1989) Changing social behaviour. The Place of Holding Communication 23: 35–39

Rimland B (1988) Physical exercise and autism. Autism Res Rev Int 2: 3

Rimland B (1995) Studies of high dose vitamin B6 in autistic children and adults – 1965–1994. Autism Research Institute, San Diego

Rimland B (1998) The use of secretin in autism: some preliminary answers. Autism Res Rev Int 12: 3

Rimland B (2000) "Garbage science" brick walls crossword puzzles and mercury. Autism Res Rev Int 14: 3

Rimland B, Edelson SM (1994) The effects of Auditory Integration Training on autism. Am J Speech-Language Pathol 5: 16–24

Rimland B, Edelson SM (1995) Brief report: A pilot study of Auditory Integration Training in autism. J Autism Dev Disord 25: 61–70

Rogers SJ (1996) Brief Report: Early intervention in autism. J Autism Dev Disord 26: 243–246

Rogers SJ (1998) Empirically supported comprehensive treatments for young children with autism. J Clin Child Psychol 27: 168–179

Rogers SJ (2000) Interventions that facilitate socialization in children with autism. J Autism Dev Disord 30: 399–410

Rogers SJ, Ozonoff S, Maslin-Cole C (1987) An effective procedure for training early special education teams to implement a model program. J Division Early Childhood 11: 180–188

Rosenthal-Malek A, Mitchell S (1997) The effects of exercise on the self-stimulatory behaviours and positive responding of adolescents with autism. J Autism Dev Disord 27: 203–212

Rutter M (1972) Childhood schizophrenia reconsidered. J Autism Childhood Schizophr 2: 315–337

Rutter M, Bartak L (1973) Special educational treatment of autistic children: a comparative study. II. Follow-up findings and implications for services. J Child Psychol Psychiatry 14: 241–270

Sansosti FJ, Powell-Smith KA, Kincaid D (2004) A research synthesis of social story interventions for children with autism spectrum disorders. Focus Autism Other Dev Disabil 19: 194–204

Schopler E (1997) Implementation of TEACCH philosophy. In: Cohen DJ, Volkmar FR (eds) Handbook of autism and pervasive developmental disorders, 2nd edn. John Wiley, New York, pp 767–798

Schopler E, Mesibov GB (eds) (1995) Learning and cognition in autism. Plenum Press, New York

Schreibman L (2000) Intensive behavioral/psychoeducational treatments for autism: research needs and future directions. J Autism Dev Disord 30: 373–378

Seltzer MM, Krauss MW, Shattuck PT, Orsmond G, Swe A, Lord C (2003) The symptoms of autism spectrum disorders in adolescence and adulthood. J Autism Dev Disord 33: 565–581

Shea V (2004) A perspective on the research literature related to early intensive behavioural intervention (Lovaas) for young children with autism. Autism 8: 349–367

Sheinkopf SJ, Siegel B (1998) Home-based behavioral treatment for young children with autism. J Autism Dev Disord 28: 15–23

Shields J (2001) The NAS Early Bird Programme: partnership with parents in early intervention. Autism: Int J Res Pract 5: 49–56

Simpson RL, Myles BS (1993) Successful integration of children and youth with autism in mainstreamed settings. Focus Autistic Behav 7: 1–13

Sinha Y, Silove N, Wheeler D, Williams K (2004) Auditory integration training and other sound therapies for autism spectrum disorders. Cochrane Database of Systematic Reviews 1 CD 003681

Stehli A (1992) The sound of a miracle: a child's triumph over autism. Fourth Estate Publications, USA

Stone WL, Yoder PJ (2001) Predicting spoken language level in children with autism spectrum disorders. Autism: Int J Res Pract 5: 341–361

Strain PS, Hoyson M (2000) On the need for longitudinal intensive social skill intervention: LEAP follow-up outcomes for children as a case in point. Topics Early Childhood Spec Educ 20: 116–122

Sussman F (1999) More than words. The Hanen Program, Toronto

Szurck S, Berlin I (1956) Elements of psychotherapeutics with the schizophrenic child and his parents. Psychiatry 19: 1–19

The Times (July 26th 2000) Law Report: The Family Division In re D (a child) Evidence: Facilitated Communication

Tincani M (2004) Comparing the picture exchange communication system and sign language training for children with autism. Focus Autism Other Dev Disabil 19: 152–163

Tjus T, Heimann M, Nelson KE (2001) Interaction patterns between children and their teachers when using a specific multimedia and communication strategy: observations from children with autism and mixed handicaps. Autism: Int J Res Pract 5: 175–187

Trevarthen C, Aitken K, Papoudi D, Roberts JM (1998) Children with autism: diagnosis and interventions to meet their needs. Jessica Kingsley, London

Ullman LP, Krasner L (eds) (1965) Case studies in behaviour modification. Holt Rinehart and Winston, New York

Welch M (1988) Holding time. Century Hutchinson, London

Wing L (1981) Asperger's syndrome: a clinical account. Psychol Med 11: 115–129

Zappella M (1988) Il legame genitore-bambino come base della terapia dei bambini autistici. In: De Giacomo P, Scacella M (eds) Terapie dell'autismo. Ed Scientifi, Bari

Author's address: Prof. P. Howlin, Department of Community Health Sciences, St. George's Hospital Medical School, Tooting, London SW17 ORE, United Kingdom, e-mail: phowlin@ sgul.ac.uk

Schizophrenia and related disorders in children and adolescents

H. Remschmidt and **F. M. Theisen**

Department of Child and Adolescent Psychiatry, Philipps-University,
Marburg, Germany

Summary. This paper reviews the concept and recent studies on childhood and adolescent psychoses with special reference to schizophrenia. After a short historical introduction, the definition, classification, and epidemiology of child- and adolescent-onset psychoses are described, pointing out that some early-onset psychotic states seem to be related to schizophrenia (such as infantile catatonia) and others not (such as desintegrative disorder).

The frequency of childhood schizophrenia is less than 1 in 10,000 children, but there is a remarkable increase in frequency between 13 and 18 years of age. Currently, schizophrenia is diagnosed according to ICD-10 and DSM-IV criteria. The differential diagnosis includes autism, desintegrative disorder, multiplex complex developmental disorder (MCDD) respectively multiple developmental impairment (MDI), affective psychoses, Asperger syndrome, drug-induced psychosis and psychotic states caused by organic disorders.

With regard to etiology, there is strong evidence for the importance of genetic factors and for neurointegrative deficits preceding the onset of the disorder.

Treatment is based upon a multimodal approach including antipsychotic medication (mainly by atypical neuroleptics), psychotherapeutic measures, family-oriented measures, and specific measures of rehabilitation applied in about 30% of the patients after completion of inpatient treatment.

The long-term course of childhood- and adolescent-onset schizophrenia is worse than in adulthood schizophrenia, and the patients with manifestation of the disorder below the age of 14 have a very poor prognosis.

Definition, classification and epidemiology

Schizophrenic psychoses in childhood are important, but rare disorders within the spectrum of psychoses. They become increasingly common during adolescence, and the symptomatology with age becomes increasingly similar to disorders in adults. After Kraepelin (1893) first described dementia praecox and Bleuler (1911) introduced the term "schizophrenia", Homburger (1926) asserted the existence of childhood schizophrenia in his classic textbook and described some characteristic features of the disorder, including those today known as "negative symptoms".

Kanner (1943) and Asperger (1944) differentiated the meanwhile well-known autistic syndromes (early infantile autism and autistic personality disorder, now called Asperger syndrome) from the pool of childhood psychoses. Finally, Karl Leonhard (1986) has to be mentioned who delineated in his well-known book "Aufteilung der endogenen Psychosen und ihre differenzierte Ätiologie" a very early-onset type of schizophrenia which he called "infantile catatonia". Unlike many other authors, he subdivided the schizophrenic disorders into "unsystematic and systematic" schizophrenias. According to his classification, unsystematic schizophrenias are characterized by primarily affective symptoms (e.g. extreme anxiety states, delusions, hallucinations, ideas of reference) with an acute, sometimes periodic course and periods of good remission. They have more in common with affective psychoses than with the group of systematic schizophrenias, whereas systematic schizophrenias show predominantly cognitive disturbances and disturbances of voluntary functions. Their course is generally chronic, without recovery to former cognitive levels, and the prognosis is poor.

The special form of childhood schizophrenia "infantile catatonia" is characterized by motor symptoms, absent or poor language development, circumscribed intellectual impairments, negativism, a periodic course, and a

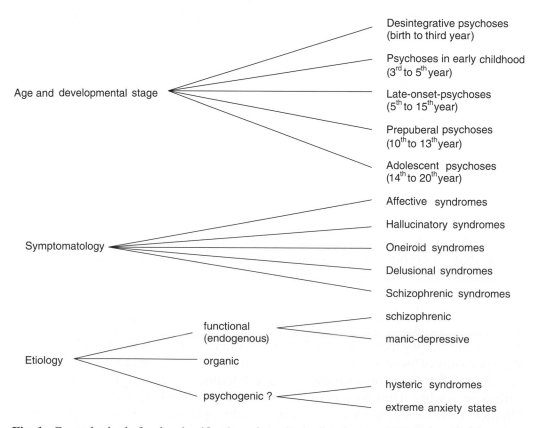

Fig. 1. General criteria for the classification of psychotic disorders in childhood and adolescence

dominance among males. To our knowledge, there is so far no study that has replicated Karl Leonhard's results regarding early infantile catatonia.

Figure 1 contains general criteria for the classification of psychotic disorders in childhood and adolescence. Classification by etiological principles would be the best method, but current knowledge does not allow reliable classifications on such a basis. Current classification systems are therefore mainly based on the symptoms of the different disorders. In childhood and adolescence, however, age and developmental stage seem to constitute an equally valid basis for classification.

The figure exemplifies three principles of classification: age and developmental stage, symptomatology and etiology. As far as etiology is concerned, it can be questioned if a psychogenic etiology (the term "reactive psychosis" is also used) does actually exist. This type of etiology has been discussed in the Scandinavian literature to some extent (Hansen et al., 1992). The clinician may come across extreme anxiety states and hysterical syndromes that show the intensity and features of acute psychotic states, but do not follow the course of schizophrenic disorders (Modestin et al., 2001). That is the reason for the question mark in Fig. 1 concerning a psychogenic etiology.

Most researchers agree that, with regard to age and developmental stage, at least four groups of psychoses in childhood and adolescence can be differentiated.

This subdivision is demonstrated in Table 1.

The *first group* of psychoses comprises various psychotic syndromes, characterized by gradual onset, chronic course, and manifestation before the third year of age. None of these psychotic syndromes, with the exception of early infantile catatonia, has any connection with schizophrenia. It has to be mentioned that some decades ago, autism was included in the category of psychotic states. This is no more the case, autism, atypical autism, and Asperger syndrome (in former times: autistic psychopathy) are now classified as "pervasive developmental disorders".

The *second group* embraces psychotic states, most of them with an acute onset between the third and fifth year of life and featuring regressive behaviour of various kinds. Their connection with schizophrenia is questionable, again with the probable exception of early infantile catatonia.

The *third group* of psychoses is characterized by an onset between late childhood and prepuberty, a fluctuating or subacute course and a clear relationship to schizophrenia of adolescence and adulthood. This applies especially to the prepubertal schizophrenia (Stutte, 1969; Eggers, 1973). The term "prepubertal schizophrenia" is no more in use today, as in the studies that propagated this term, the pubertal stages were not registered. According to Werry (1992), a distinction can be made between early-onset schizophrenia beginning in childhood or adolescence (before the age of 16 or 17) and very early-onset schizophrenia (before the age of 13). Werry separates the latter group, because that definition is more precise than the term "prepubertal". As the age of puberty varies and most studies that used the term "prepubertal schizophrenia" did not consider the pubertal stages, Werry states further that a review of the studies of childhood schizophrenia is complicated. In addition, in studies before the

Table 1. Different psychotic syndromes in childhood and adolescents and their relationship to schizophrenia (adapted from Remschmidt, 1988)

Clinical syndrome	Age at manifestation and course	Relation to schizophrenia
Group 1 (Anthony, 1958, 1962) Autism (Kanner, 1943) Pseudodefective psychosis (Bender, 1947, 1959) "No-onset" type (Despert, 1938)	Early manifestation until third year of life and chronic course	No relation to schizophrenia
Early infantile catatonia (Leonhard, 1986)	Manifestation before third year of life possible	Relation to schizophrenia likely
Group 2 (Anthony, 1958, 1962) Dementia infantilis (Heller, 1908) Dementia praecocissima (DeSanctis, 1908) Pseudoneurotic schizophrenia (Bender, 1947, 1959) "Acute-onset" type (Despert, 1938) Symbiotic psychosis (Mahler et al., 1949; Mahler, 1952) Asperger syndrome (Asperger, 1944, 1968)	Manifestation between third and fifth year of life with acute course and regressive behavior	Relation to schizophrenia questionable
Early infantile catatonia (Leonhard, 1986)	Most frequent manifestation within the first 6 years of life	Relation to schizophrenia likely
Group 3 (Anthony, 1958, 1962) Psychoses (late-onset psychoses) (Kolvin, 1971) Pseudopsychopathic schizophrenia (Bender, 1959)	Late-onset psychoses (late childhood and prepuberty) with fluctuating, subacute course	Relation to schizophrenia of adolescence and also adulthood (Anthony, 1958, 1962; Eisenberg, 1957; Rimland, 1964; Rutter, 1967)
Prepuberal schizophrenia (Stutte, 1969; Eggers, 1973)	Manifestation in prepuberty	Clear relation to schizophrenia
Group 4 Adolescent schizophrenia	Manifestation during prepuberty	Clear relation to schizophrenia

introduction of ICD-9 and DSM-III, many psychotic disorders of childhood were aggregated into the single category "childhood schizophrenia". So in many articles, it is impossible to differentiate between early infantile autism, childhood schizophrenia and other psychotic states of childhood.

The *fourth group* of psychoses is formed by adolescent schizophrenia which manifests at puberty and adolescence and is clearly related to schizophrenia. Psychoses manifested during adolescence may or may not have precursor symptoms in childhood (Rutter, 1967; Remschmidt, 1975a, b). This subdivision according to premorbid personality and psychosocial adaptation also seems to be important in positive and negative schizophrenia in adolescents, because there is a relationship between poor premorbid adjustment and negative symptoms in schizophrenia in adulthood (Andreasen and Olsen, 1982) as well as during adolescence (Remschmidt et al., 1991).

The concept of positive and negative symptoms of schizophrenia in children and adolescents

The concept of positive and negative symptoms in schizophrenia has been widely employed and supported in general psychiatry. It can, however, also be applied to childhood and adolescent schizophrenia (Bettes and Walker, 1987; Remschmidt et al., 1994).

Bettes and Walker (1987) studied a sample of 1,084 children in whom psychosis had been diagnosed. For all patients, the presence or absence of 31 symptoms, including psychotic symptoms, was recorded at intake by a psychiatrist, a psychologist, and a social worker. The investigators found that the manifestation of positive and negative symptoms was strongly affected by age. Positive symptoms increased linearly with age, while negative symptoms were most frequent in early childhood and later adolescence. This was the case both for the total sample of children and for the subsample of children with psychotic diagnoses. There were only a few differences between males and females with regard to symptoms. A further finding was a correlation between symptomatology and intelligence quotient: Children with high IQ's showed more positive and fewer negative symptoms than children with low IQ's. This investigation underlines the notion suggested by earlier studies that age and developmental stage are decisive for symptomatology of psychotic states in childhood, as stated in Table 1.

Remschmidt et al. (1994) studied a sample of 61 schizophrenic patients subdivided into two groups. Group I comprised 11 patients with first manifestation of schizophrenia before the age of 14, group II 40 patients with first manifestation of the disorder after the age of 14. To get information about positive and negative symptoms and other precursors of schizophrenia, the Instrument for the Retrospective Assessment of the Onset of Schizophrenia (IRAOS) was administered. IRAOS is a semi-structured interview that allows the retrospective assessment of schizophrenia and other symptoms before the first manifestation of the disorder. This instrument was developed by Häfner and his group (Häfner et al., 1990) and modified by our group for the investigation of children and adolescents and their parents. It could be demonstrated that negative as well

Table 2. Comparison of the ICD-10 and DSM-IV classification of schizophrenia and related disorders

Schizophrenia, schizotypical and delusional disorders (ICD-10)	Schizophrenia and other psychotic disorders (DSM-IV)
Schizophrenia	Schizophrenia
Paranoid schizophrenia	Paranoid type
Hebephrenic schizophrenia	Disorganized type
Catatonic schizophrenia	Catatonic type
Undifferentiated schizophrenia	Undifferentiated type
Post-schizophrenic depression	
Residual schizophrenia	Residual type
Simple schizophrenia	
Classification of course possible	Classification of course possible
Schizotypical disorder	Schizophreniform disorder
Persistent delusional disorder	Delusional disorder
Acute and transient psychotic disorder	Brief psychotic disorder
Induced delusional disorder	Shared psychotic disorder (folie à deux)
Schizoaffective disorder with subtype: manic, depressive and mixed	Schizoaffective disorder: bipolar subtype, depressive subtype
	Psychotic disorder due to a general medical condition
	Substance-induced psychotic disorder

as positive symptoms appear in both groups a long time before the clinical manifestation of the disorder which led to admission. While many patients showed both negative and positive symptoms before the index admission, both categories of symptoms become more frequent and converge at the time of the admission.

Table 2 shows a comparison of schizophrenia and other psychotic disorders according to the two classification systems ICD-10 and DSM-IV.

As the table demonstrates, many categories correspond with one another in both systems. There are, however, some differences. These concern the sub-types of schizophrenia and the inclusion of psychotic disorders due to general medical conditions and in substance-induced psychotic disorders. These disorders are classified in ICD-10 under other categories.

The *schizophreniform* disorder in DSM-IV is somewhat different as compared to schizotypical disorder in ICD-10. The diagnosis of schizophreniform disorder requires the identical criteria of schizophrenia, except for two differences: The total duration of the illness is at least one month, but less than six months, and impaired social or occupational functioning during some part of the illness is not required. There are also some other differences; however, they are less important for childhood and adolescent schizophrenia.

A major query is, however, that the diagnosis schizophrenia according to DSM-IV requires a duration of six months, whereas in ICD-10 a duration of only one month is required. With regard to these differences, some disorders may be diagnosed as schizophrenia according to ICD-10 criteria, but not to those of DSM-IV.

In spite of the fact that childhood and adolescent schizophrenia lie on a continuum with adult schizophrenia, there are special difficulties in applying the "adult criteria" to younger children with suspected schizophrenia. Symptoms at an early age are less specific and show remarkable overlap with a number of developmental disorders. This leads to a greater uncertainty regarding the diagnosis especially in younger children. This uncertainty can lead to the desire to confirm the diagnosis over a period of time which in turn can result in the loss of valuable time for early treatment. Recent research suggests that early treatment seems to improve the outcome especially with the new atypical neuroleptics.

Epidemiology

In general, there is agreement that schizophrenia is a severe psychiatric disorder even in childhood and adolescence. The lifetime prevalence of schizophrenia is approximately 1%. It is assumed that only 0.1 to 1% of all schizophrenic psychoses manifest themselves before the age of 10 and 70% of all schizophrenic disorders occur between the age of 20 and 45. In the general population, approximately one child in 10,000 will develop a schizophrenic disorder (Remschmidt et al., 1994). There are a few epidemiological studies which are able to confront questions of frequency, age and sex distribution, treatment and course of child and adolescent schizophrenia. Werry (1992) states that the results of studies carried out before 1975 are questionable, because at this time, no internationally accepted classification schemes were available. According to several authors, however, the following statements can be forwarded: The prevalence rate of very early-onset schizophrenia (manifestation before the age of 12) is less than one child in 10,000 children between 2 and 12 years of age (Burd and Kerbeshian, 1987). It is estimated that childhood-onset schizophrenia is approximately 50 times less frequent than adult-onset schizophrenia, it is also less frequent than autism. There is a remarkable increase of schizophrenia after the 13th year of life (Remschmidt et al., 1994).

Diagnosis and differential diagnosis

Diagnostic procedures

Psychotic disorders, especially schizophrenic disorders in children and adolescents, are normally diagnosed according to the criteria of ICD-10 and DSM-IV. Usually, the diagnosis is based upon a careful history of the patient and his family taken from the parents and the patient himself and a thorough clinical investigation of the patient, including psychological respectively neuropsychological testing. The test psychological investigation should include cognitive measures on intelligence, concentration, memory, language, and motor functions. In addition, it is very important to include also measures covering the emotional state of the patient. Depressive symptoms are frequently either precursors or a common trait in the beginning of adolescent schizophrenia. Approximately 20% of adolescents with schizophrenia start the disorder with a depressive episode (Remschmidt et al., 1973).

Table 3. Instruments for the diagnosis of schizophrenic disorders in childhood and adolescence

Clinical Interviews		
K-SADS-E	Parents/Child	6–17 y.
(Schedule for Affective Disorder and Schizophrenia for School-Age Children)		
ICDS	Parents/Child	6–18 y.
(Interview for Childhood Disorders and Schizophrenia)		
CAPA	Parents/Child	8–18 y.
(Child and Adolescent Psychiatric Assessment)		
DICA	Parents/Child	6–17 y.
(Diagnostic Interview for Children and Adolescents)		
NJMH DISC	Parents/Child	9–17 y.
Scales		
KIDDIE-PANSS	Interviewer Parents/Child	6–16 y.
CPRS	Interviewer/Child	up to 15 y.
(Children's Psychiatric Rating Scale)		
TDS	Child	5–13 y.
(Thought-Disorder-Scales)		

There exist also more or less standardized clinical interviews and scales for the diagnosis of schizophrenia during childhood and adolescence mostly used for research purposes. The most frequently used instruments are summarized in Table 3.

Differential diagnosis

There are several disorders that have to be distinguished from schizophrenia during the age of childhood and adolescence. They are discussed in the following.

(1) Autism

Autism is now looked upon as a pervasive developmental disorder with manifestation in the first 30 months of life with a characteristic symptomatology that differs from schizophrenia, but has several symptoms in common. Hallucinations and delusions, however, are not found in autism and such an early onset of the disorder is not found in schizophrenia. In most cases, the differential diagnosis can be based upon the history taken from the parents, clinical observation, and the course of the disorder. There might be only one psychotic state which might be difficult to differentiate from schizophrenia: This is the early infantile catatonia, described by Karl Leonhard (1986). To date, it is not clear if this disorder is really the first manifestation of schizophrenia or if some of Leonhard's cases could be looked upon as a kind of atypical autism.

(2) Desintegrative disorder (Heller's syndrome)

This syndrome is characterized by a normal development until the age of 3 or 4, followed by a progressive deterioration and the loss of already acquired abilities.

The syndrome is very rare as compared to autism and also less frequent than early onset schizophrenia. Characteristic is the loss of already acquired functions, including language, together with characteristic abnormalities of social, communicative and behavioural functioning. The children become frequently irritable, anxious, and overactive before the full clinical picture becomes apparent. There are again at least two distinct criteria by which this disorder can be distinguished from schizophrenia:

– the early loss of acquired skills and
– the early onset of the disorder.

(3) Multiplex complex developmental disorders (MCDD), respectively multiple developmental impairment (MDI)

These disorders are not yet included in the ICD-10 or DSM-IV classification systems, respectively.

MCDD was first described by Towbin et al. (1993) as a syndrome characterized by "disturbances in affect modulation, social relatedness and thinking", whereas MDI (McKenna et al., 1994) is a label for children who are characterized by brief transient psychotic symptoms, age-inappropriate phantasies, and magical thinking which cannot be clearly looked upon as a delusional phenomenon, social withdrawal, emotional lability, and deficits in information processing. The criteria for childhood schizophrenia are not fulfilled, and the major difference between schizophrenic children and MDI children is twofold: They reveal less negative symptoms and are less socially impaired.

The two syndromes MCDD and MDI are overlapping to a certain extent. Whereas the MCDD construct seems to be closer to the concept of pervasive developmental disorders, the MDI concept seems to have a greater affinity to schizophrenia. The relationship of both syndromes to schizophrenia is not completely clear, however, a follow-up study on MCDD children demonstrated that approximately 20% developed schizophrenia later on in their lives (van der Gaag, 1993).

A follow-up study of 19 MDI patients, however, did not confirm this development. So the question arises if this syndrome is a precursor syndrome of schizophrenia (Jacobsen and Rapoport, 1998).

(4) Affective psychoses (psychotic depression, bipolar disorder)

As already stated earlier in this article, adolescent schizophrenia often starts with a depressive episode. On the other hand, there are studies that demonstrate that bipolar disorders are very often initially diagnosed as schizophrenia (Werry et al., 1991).

In most cases, however, a differentiation is possible during the first half year of observation. This can be done by the typical symptom clusters that are different between schizophrenia and bipolar disorder.

(5) Asperger syndrome

The leading features that allow to differentiate Asperger's disorder from schizophrenia are the individual history of the patient (symptoms of autistic spectrum disorder, very early language acquisition), the clinical observation and the course. As far as the clinical picture is concerned, patients with Asperger syndrome usually do not reveal positive symptoms and a deterioration of their scholastic and social functioning is missing. It is, however, known that some cases of Asperger syndrome may develop schizophrenia later on in life (Wolff, 1995).

(6) Drug-induced psychosis

This may be to date the most frequent differential diagnosis. Many adolescents who come to clinical attendance with a psychotic state have consumed drugs, and it is difficult to decide if the clinical picture represents schizophrenia or a psychotic state caused by organic brain conditions. And even if the clinical symptomatology fulfils the criteria of schizophrenia, the question arises if the disorder was caused by the consumed substances or only triggered. There are many drugs that are known to induce psychotic states (Marihuana, LSD, Cocaine, amphetamines, alcohol hypnotics, anxiolytics). The differentiation from schizophrenia can be done by a thorough history taking including an inquiry about all substances taken during the last year and by laboratory investigations. The diagnosis of schizophrenia can be confirmed if the symptoms persist for several months after drug withdrawal.

(7) Organic brain disorders

There are several organic brain disorders that are known to be associated with psychotic states, among them temporal epilepsy and some neurodegenerative disorders such as Morbus Wilson, Chorea Huntington and Juvenile Metachromatic Leucodystrophia. These disorders can be detected and delineated from schizophrenia by thorough neurological examinations including laboratory tests. The clinical picture very often is characterized by movement disorders and a progressive deterioration of cognitive functions.

Etiology

In 2002, we summarized the major etiological components in child and adolescent schizophrenia (Remschmidt, 2002). The major etiological components comprise genetic findings, neurobiological and neuropsychological results. These are demonstrated in Table 4.

As far as genetic results are concerned, family studies, twin and adoption studies demonstrate very clearly the importance of genetic influences (for review, see Schourfield and McGuffin, 2001). Molecular genetic studies have identified several replicated candidate gene regions. We are, however, still far away from a convincing genetic explanation of the disorder. It can be assumed that schizophrenia is a complex disorder caused by quite a number of genes and also influenced to a considerable extent by environmental factors.

There are interesting biological and neuropsychological results with regard to early-onset schizophrenia as summarized in Table 4, and it is

Table 4. Components concerning the etiology of schizophrenia in childhood and adolescence

1. Genetic results (all in adult patients): 6 replicated candidate gene regions on the chromosomes 6, 8, 10, 13, 18, 22

2. Neurobiological results:

• Brain morphology:	Reduction of the total cerebral volume, correlation with negative symptoms
• Biochemical studies:	Abnormalities in the glutamatergic, dopaminergic, serotonergic and noradrenergic system
• Electrophysiological studies:	Skin conductance: high baseline activity, slow habituation evoked potentials: controversial results

3. Neuropsychological results:

• Cognitive impairment:	IQ↓, attention deficits, reduced language perception, disturbances in the organisation of perception
• Neurointegrative deficits:	Pandysmaturation (PDM) (Fish, 1975)
• Attention deficits:	Are they correlated with deficits in understanding social relationships?
• Communication deficits:	Poor speech production, incoherent language, unclear and ambiguous way of referring to their surroundings, formal thought disorders

evident that the developmental perspective contributes much to the current understanding of schizophrenic disorders (Remschmidt, 2002). Examples for that can be given from the field of biochemistry and neuropsychology. There are for instance developmental changes of the glutamatergic system during adolescence (in animal studies) as a sensitization of adolescent rat brain to glutamate antagonists (e.g. phencyclidine) and a dysfunction of the N-methyl-D-aspartate (NDMA)-receptor (Keshevan and Hogarty, 1999) which might be responsible for the causation of psychotic states by the glutamate antagonist phencyclidine during adolescence in clinical context, a well-known phenomenon.

In terms of neurodevelopmental deficits the concept of pandysmaturation (PDM) has raised great attention. PDM (Fish, 1975) stands for a neurointegrative deficit operationalized by three criteria: (1) Transient retardation of motor and/or visual motor development, (2) abnormal profile of function on a developmental examination and (3) accompanied by a retardation of sceletal growth. There are several studies (Fish et al., 1992; Done et al., 1994; Jones et al., 1994; Hollis, 2003) that replicated a delayed development in children of schizophrenic parents and pre-schizophrenics and certain developmental delays seem to be a precursor of early-onset schizophrenia. In addition, IQ-decline during childhood (between ages 4 and 7) was predictive of psychotic symptoms but not of other psychiatric symptoms at age 23 (Kremen et al., 1998).

The very early-onset schizophrenia seems to be somewhat different from the schizophrenic disorders with manifestation during adolescence or later. In our view, very early-onset schizophrenia can be looked upon as a progressive-deteriorating developmental disorder (Remschmidt, 2002), and there are four arguments for this view:

– Increasing ventricular volume during the course of the disorder and progressive loss of cerebellar volume (Keller et al., 2003; Rapoport et al., 1997). But also in adolescence progressive gray matter loss was found to be specific to schizophrenia (Gogtay et al., 2003).
– deterioration of intellectual functioning during the course of the disorder (Jacobsen and Rapoport, 1998),
– extremely unfavourable outcome which is worse than in adolescent-onset and adult-onset schizophrenia (Remschmidt et al., 2005),
– shift from positive symptoms to negative symptoms beginning during inpatient treatment and becoming stable during the long-term course (Remschmidt et al., 1994, 2005).

Treatment and rehabilitation

There are at least four components that are important for treatment and rehabilitation in child and adolescent schizophrenia: Treatment with neuroleptics, psychotherapeutic measures, family-oriented measures, and specific measures of rehabilitation.

Treatment with neuroleptics

As in adult psychiatry, currently atypical neuroleptics are mainly used that are characterized by the following properties:

– A different receptor-binding profile as compared to conventional neuroleptics (lower binding to dopamine receptors, higher affinity to 5-HT$_{2A}$ and $\alpha 1$ receptors) which is responsible for a different action,
– a low rate of extrapyramidal side effects (EPS) as a consequence of this receptor-binding profile,
– efficacy also with regard to negative symptoms in contrast to most conventional neuroleptics, and
– absence of hyperprolactinaemia and a low rate of other adverse effects.

Table 5 gives an overview of the most frequently used antipsychotic (neuroleptic) medications and Fig. 2 demonstrates a decision tree for the selection of antipsychotics in childhood and adolescent schizophrenia.

The psychopharmacological treatment has at least three foci: Management of acute psychotic states, prevention of relapses, and controlling the side effects.

Acute psychotic states normally require an inpatient treatment during which antipsychotic drugs play a predominant role. Currently, treatment will be started with an atypical antipsychotic drug in case of severe agitation and aggressive outbursts, a benzodiazepine or a typical moderate or low potency neuroleptic (e.g. levomepromazine) can be used additionally. The further strategy of pharmacological treatment can be applied according to the algorithm displayed in Fig. 2. Depending on the individual reaction (efficacy and side

Table 5. Most frequently used antipsychotic medications in child and adolescent schizophrenia

	Sedation	Positive symptoms	Negative symptoms	Neuroleptic potency	Usual oral dose (usual depot dose i.m.)
Typical high potency neuroleptics					
Benperidol	+	++	++	100	1–6 mg/dy
Flupenthixol (-decanoate)	+	++	++	50	2–10 mg/dy (20–100 mg/2–4 weeks)
Fluphenazine (-decanoate)	+(+)	+++	++	30	5–20 mg/day (12.5–100 mg/2–4 weeks)
Fluspirilene	+	+++	++	300	(2–10 mg/week)[a]
Haloperidol (-decanoate)	+	+++	++	60	2–20 mg/day (50–300 mg/2–4 weeks)
Perphenazine (-enanthate)	++	+++	++	8	12–64 mg/day (50–200 mg/2 weeks)
Pimozide	+	+++	++	50	4–20 mg/day
Typical moderate and low potency neuroleptics					
Chlorpromazine	+++	+++	++	1	150–600 mg/day
Chlorprothixene	+++	++	+++	0.8	150–600 mg/day
Levomepromazine	+++	++	+++	0.8	75–600 mg/day
Perazine	++	++	++	0.5	75–600 mg/day
Pipamperone	+++			0.2	120–360 mg/day
Promethazine	+++				50–400 mg/day
Sulpiride	+	++	+++	0.5	100–800 mg/day
Thioridazine	+++	++	++	0.7	200–700 mg/day
Tiapride	+				300–600 mg/day
Atypical neuroleptics					
Amisulpride	+	+++	+++		50–400 mg/day[1] / 400–800 mg/day[2]
Aripiprazole	+	+++	+++		10–30 mg/day
Clozapine	+++	+++	+++	(0.5–2)	25–600 mg/day
Olanzapine	++	+++	+++	(8–20)	10–20 mg/day
Quetiapine	+	+++	+++		150–750 mg/day
Risperidone (Risperdal Consta®) 25/37.5/50 mg][b]	+	+++	+++	(50)	1–12 mg/day (25–50 mg/2 weeks)
Ziprasidone	++	+++	+++		80–160 mg/day
Zotepine	++	+++	+++	(2)	75–300 mg/day

+ = none or low, ++ = moderate, +++ = high. [a] Available only as depot neuroleptic, [b] currently the only atypical depot neuroleptic (in Germany available since July 2002). [1] for patients with predominantly negative symptoms, [2] for patients with predominantly positive symptoms

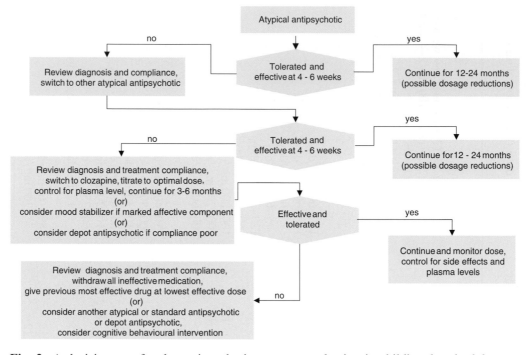

Fig. 2. A decision tree for the antipsychotic treatment selection in childhood and adolescent schizophrenia (adapted and modified from Clark and Lewis, 1998)

effects), the decisions for switching or maintaining the present medication are made. In most countries, clozapine can only be initiated after two different compounds that have not proven effective or were not tolerated by the patients. The usual oral dosages, and for depot-neuroleptics the intramuscular dosages, are given in Table 5.

Prevention of relapses requires the application of a long-term antipsychotic medication. Relapses are frequently triggered by emotional stress, adverse life events, but also by positive emotional experiences. With regard to these factors, it is very important to anticipate a relapse prevention by either maintaining low-dose oral medication or by switching to a depot-neuroleptic. Especially when the compliance is a problem, a depot-medication is recommended. Currently, to our knowledge, only risperdal-consta is available as an atypic depot-neuroleptic, at least in Germany.

The third major focus is controlling of side effects. The incidence rates of extrapyramidal symptoms caused by typical neuroleptics are higher in children and adolescents than in adults. Therefore, atypical neuroleptics are usually preferred. The advantage of the atypical neuroleptics is the fact that they do not induce or have only a low risk of inducing extrapyramidal side effects. Several atypical neuroleptics, however, cause other side effects that are also a considerable strain for the patients, among them extreme weight gain, most pronounced after the application of clozapine and olanzapine. Therefore, recently new compounds have been developed with a lower risk of weight gain such as aripiprazole. To date, however, there are only a few experiences in the treatment of childhood and adolescent-onset schizophrenia. Especially, during adolescence, weight gain is one of the most frequent causes of non-compliance. There are several other adverse effects related to different types of antipsychotics which cannot be described in detail here (for review, see Remschmidt et al., 2001).

Psychotherapeutic measures

Psychotherapeutic treatment includes at least four components:

(1) A careful and comprehensive information about the disorder within the psychoeducational approach,
(2) cognitive psychotherapy and other behavioural measures,
(3) emotional management therapy, and
(4) group programmes.

The *information about the disorder* is essential and should include also the family. All explanations have to be adapted to the phase of the disorder and the cognitive and emotional level of the patient.

Psychotherapeutic measures based on *cognitive interventions* include different strategies such as distraction treatment, rationale responding, belief modification, and the enhancement of coping strategies. The aim of all these treatment approaches is to give the patient an active role and to enhance his specific abilities to cope with symptoms of the disorder, distress and anxiety. There exist integrated approaches based on several components. One of these, successfully applied to adolescent schizophrenia, is the "Integrative Psychological Therapy Programme for Schizophrenic Patients (IPT)" developed in Switzerland (Brenner et al., 1980, 1993). This programme consists of five standardized therapeutic components: Cognitive differentiation, social perception, verbal communication, social skills, and interpersonal problem solving. The programme started originally from the classical social skills training technique, which was extended to the area of communication. It is possible to administer the programme individually to patients with a different profile of schizophrenic symptoms. Most of the tasks of this programme, assigned to the different therapy components, are realistic and orientated towards everyday situations and can be offered in the form of slides and video sequences. This programme, originally developed for young adults, has been modified for adolescents (Kienzle et al., 1997) and seems to offer a promising approach that still needs to be evaluated systematically.

Emotional management therapy so far has not yet been demonstrated to be effective in young patients with schizophrenia; however, there is no doubt that the emotional sphere is of great importance in the course of the disorder. But studies are needed that evaluate the effect of this approach. *Group programmes* have been thought to be helpful in the treatment of young patients with schizophrenia and have been applied with the main focus on the improvement of skills (e.g. social skills training, problem-solving, communication) and education (e.g. information about illness and treatment, management of medication and relapses). The already mentioned IPT-programme has frequently and successfully been applied as a group programme.

Family-oriented measures

It is evident that the families of children and adolescents with schizophrenia have to be included in the planning and the concept of treatment. However, empirical research has shown that ambitious family therapy concepts which have been propagated in the last decades have not brought the benefits hoped for. It is now quite clear that the "typical psychotic family" does not exist nor the "schizophrenogenic mother". On the other hand, the concept of expressed emotions is an important one and demonstrates the important role of the family with regard to relapses of the disorder. Therefore, in every case of child and adolescent schizophrenia, one has to decide to which extent the family should be integrated into the therapeutic process. This depends largely on the patient, the disorder, the structure and stability of the family, as well as the therapist's experience. There are the following components that can be included in the family-oriented approaches in the treatment of schizophrenia (Remschmidt et al., 2001):

- Family counselling and psychoeducational approaches:
  The main aim of this type of intervention is the development of a stable therapeutic alliance comprising detailed information about the disorder, measures of treatment, and information about course and prognosis. Special emphasis has to be laid on medication, including the most important effects and side effects and the different components used.
- Supportive and structural family therapy:
  Within this approach, the major aim is the neutralization and control of symptoms. This means that secondary problems, conflicts and vicious circles which frequently develop in the course of the psychotic disorder need to be interrupted. While the first level of family interventions (family counselling) is carried out individually with parents on one side and with the patient on the other side, supportive and structural family therapy is carried out during joint sessions in which both parents and the patient actively take part, sometimes also with siblings and other family members. However, this kind of intervention is only possible when a significant reduction of symptoms has already taken place and a good cooperation with the family has been achieved.
- Extended development-oriented family therapy:
  This third level of family intervention can only be carried out in a minority of families with a psychotic child or adolescent. The main focus is concentrated on the pattern of relationship between the family members and typical family conflicts which inhibit the patient's development. This type of intervention requires very experienced therapists, cooperative families and can be used only in rare cases.

Specific measures of rehabilitation

Approximately 40% of children and adolescents with schizophrenia are not able to continue on their prepsychotic level regarding school, professional work, communication, and social integration. For these patients, residential rehabilitation may be indicated because of either the nature or the course of their illness. Especially in patients with marked negative symptoms after treatment of their acute episode, a re-integration into the family might not be possible. For these patients, a programme has been developed with the Department of Child and Adolescent Psychiatry of the Philipps-University of Marburg and the rehabilitation center "Leppermuehle" near Marburg. This rehabilitation programme is on average of 2-years' duration and includes the following components (Martin, 1991; Remschmidt et al., 2001):

(1) A well-structured educational facility with expertise in dealing with particular special needs of these adolescents.
(2) As an integral component of the rehabilitation process helping the adolescents to realize their educational capacity, with the acquisition of relevant qualifications.
(3) Individual supportive psychotherapy and additional group work involving social skills training.
(4) Occupational therapy as an important rehabilitation measure and, for older adolescents, integration into appropriate work activities.
(5) Finally, individually tailored medication in order to minimize the risk of relapse.

These general principles have been realized in an integrated rehabilitation programme. The major components of this programme are demonstrated in Fig. 3.

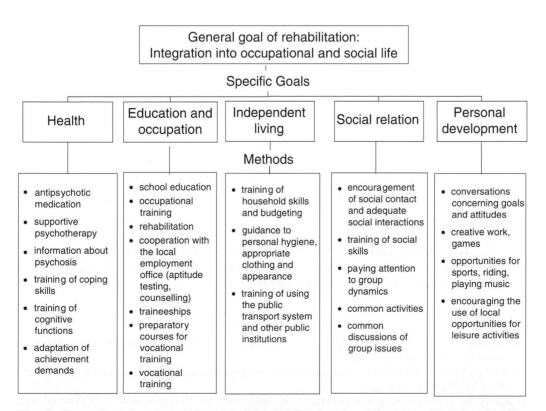

Fig. 3. General goal and specific goals of rehabilitation in adolescent schizophrenia after inpatient treatment

138   H. Remschmidt and F. M. Theisen

As Fig. 3 demonstrates, there are five goals with regard to the integration of the patients into occupational and social life. These are: Health, education and occupation, independent living, social relations, and personal development.

The figure describes also the major methods by which these goals can be reached. For example, in order to reach and maintain health, the continuation of an antipsychotic medication is important as well as supportive psychotherapy, information about the disorder, training of coping skills and cognitive functions, and also a training to adapt to the demands of the environment in which the patient is living.

This programme has been successful in an one-year follow-up, and a further long-term evaluation is under way.

For a more detailed description of the programme, see Remschmidt et al. (2001).

Course and outcome

With regard to course and outcome, the results of the few existing studies (for review, see Merry and Werry, 2001; Fleischhaker et al., 2005) can be summarized as follows:

(1) Schizophrenic disorders with manifestation before the age of 14 have a very poor prognosis. The disorder continues in most cases to adolescence and to adulthood and can be diagnosed by the same criteria as for adults (Asarnow et al., 1994).
(2) Patients with acute manifestation of the disorder and with productive schizophrenic symptoms such as hallucinations and delusions (positive symptoms) have on average a better prognosis than those with slow manifestation, insidious course and with continuous impairment of cognitive functions and/or depressive states (Remschmidt et al., 1991).
(3) Premorbid personality is of great importance. Patients who had been described in the premorbid phase as socially active, intelligent and well-integrated children and adolescents have a better prognosis than those who had been cognitively impaired, shy, introverted and withdrawn before the manifestation of their disorder (Martin, 1991; Werry et al., 1991, 1994).
(4) Finally, the prognosis seems to be better in patients without any family load of schizophrenia, good cooperation of the family and rapid improvement during inpatient treatment (Martin, 1991; Remschmidt et al., 1991).
(5) The few course and outcome studies confirm the result that prognosis and outcome in childhood and early adolescent schizophrenia is much worse than in adult schizophrenia (Fleischhaker et al., 2005).

References

Andreasen NC, Olsen S (1982) Negative vs. positive schizophrenia: definition and validation. Arch Gen Psychiatry 39: 789–794
Anthony EJ (1958) An experimental approach to the psychopathology of childhood autism. Br J Med Psychol 31: 211–225
Anthony EJ (1962) Low-grade psychosis in childhood. In: Richards BW (ed) Proceedings, London Conference on Scientific Study of Mental Deficiency, vol 2. May and Baker, Dagenham (Essex), pp 398–410

Asarnow RF, Asamen J, Granholm E et al. (1994) Cognitive/neuropsychological studies of children with a schizophrenic disorder. Schizophr Bull 20: 647–670

Asperger H (1944) Die "autistischen Psychopathen" im Kindes- und Jugendalter. Arch Psychiatr Nervenkrankh 117: 76–136

Asperger H (1968) Zur Differentialdiagnose des kindlichen Autismus. Acta Paedopsychiatr 35: 136–146

Bender L (1947) Childhood schizophrenia: clinical study of one hundred schizophrenic children. Am J Orthopsychiatr 17: 40–56

Bender L (1959) The concept of pseudopsychopathic schizophrenia in adolescence. Am J Orthopsychiatr 29: 491–509

Bettes BA, Walker E (1987) Positive and negative symptoms in psychotic and other psychiatrically disturbed children. J Child Psychol Psychiatr Allied Disciplines 28: 555–568

Bleuler E (1911) Dementia praecox oder die Gruppe der Schizophrenien. Deuticke, Leipzig

Brenner HD, Stramke WG, Mewes J, Liese F, Seeger G (1980) Erfahrungen mit einem spezifischen Therapieprogramm zum Training kognitiver und kommunikativer Fähigkeiten in der Rehabilitation chronisch schizophrener Patienten. Nervenarzt 51: 106–112

Brenner HD, Roder V, Merlo MCG (1993) Verhaltenstherapeutische Verfahren bei schizophrenen Erkrankungen. In: Möller HJ (ed) Therapie psychiatrischer Erkrankungen. Enke, Stuttgart, pp 222–230

Burd L, Kerbeshian J (1987) A North-Dacota prevalence study of schizophrenia presenting in childhood. J Am Acad Child Adolesc Psychiatry 26: 347–350

Clark AF, Lewis SW (1998) Practitioner review: treatment of schizophrenia in childhood and adolescence. J Child Psychol Psychiatry 39: 1071–1081

DeSanctis S (1908) Dementia praecocissima catatonica. Folia Neurobiol 1: 9–12

Despert JL (1938) Schizophrenia in children. Psychiatr Quart 12: 366–371

Done DJ, Crow TJ, Johnstone EC, Sacker A (1994) Childhood antecedents of schizophrenia and affective illness: social adjustment at ages 7 and 11. Br Med J 309: 699–703

Eggers C (1973) Verlaufsweisen kindlicher und präpuberaler Schizophrenien. Springer, Berlin

Fish B (1975) Biological antecedents of psychosis in children. In: Friedmann D (ed) The biology of major psychosis. Raven Press, New York, pp 49–80

Fish B, Marcus J, Hans SL et al. (1992) Infants at risk for schizophrenia: sequelae of genetic neurointegrative deficit. Arch Gen Psychiatry 49: 221–235

Fleischhaker C, Tepper K, Hennighausen K, Schulz E, Remschmidt H (2005) Long-term course of adolescent schizophrenia. Schizophr Bull (in press)

Gogtay N, Sporn H, Nicolson R, Classen L, Greenstein D, Giedd JN, Gochman P, Lennane M, Evans A, Rapoport JL (2003) Progressive cortical gray matter loss in adolescence is specific to schizophrenia. Schizophr Res 60/1 [Suppl]: 196–196

Häfner H, Riecher A, Maurer K, Meissner S, Schmidtke A, Fätkenheuer B, Löffler W, An der Heiden W (1990) Instrument for the Retrospective Assessment of the Onset of Schizophrenia (IRAOS). Z Klin Psychol 19: 230–255

Hansen H, Dahl AA, Bertelsen A, Birket-Smith M, von Knorring L, Ottosson JO (1992) The Nordic concept of reactive psychosis – a multicenter reliability study. Acta Psychiatr Scand 86: 55–59

Heller T (1908) Über Dementia infantilis (Verblödungsprozess im Kindesalter). Z Erforschung und Behandlung des jugendlichen Schwachsinns auf wissenschaftlicher Grundlage 2: 17–28

Hollis C (2003) Develomental precursors of child- and adolescent-onset schizophrenia and affective psychoses: diagnostic specifity and continuity with symptom dimensions. Br J Psychiatry 182: 37–44

Homburger A (1926) Vorlesungen über Psychopathologie des Kindesalters. Springer, Berlin

Jacobsen LK, Rapoport JL (1998) Research update: Childhood onset schizophrenia: implications of clinical and neurobiological research. J Child Psychol Psychiatry 39: 101–113

Jones P, Rodgers B, Murray RM (1994) Child development risk factors for adult schizophrenia in the British 1946 birth cohort. Lancet 344: 1398–1402

Kanner L (1943) Autistic disturbances of affective contact. The Nervous Child 2: 217–250

Keller A, Castellanos FX, Vaituzis AC, Jeffries NO, Giedd JN, Rapoport JL (2003) Progressive loss of cerebellar volume in childhood-onset schizophrenia. Am J Psychiatry 160: 128–133

Keshavan MS, Hogarty GE (1999) Brain maturational processes and delayed onset in schizophrenia. Dev Psychopathol 11: 525–543

Kienzle N, Braun-Scharm H, Hemme M (1997) Kognitive, psychoedukative und familientherapeutische Therapiebausteine in der stationären jugendpsychiatrischen Versorgung. In: Dittmar HE, Klein E, Schön D (eds) Integrative Therapiemodelle und ihre Wirksamkeit. Roderer, Regensburg, pp 139–152

Kolvin I (1971) Studies in the childhood psychoses. I. Diagnostic criteria and classification. Br J Psychiatry 118: 381–384

Kolvin I, Garside RF, Kidd JSH (1971a) Studies in the childhood psychoses. IV. Parental personality and attitude and childhood psychosis. Br J Psychiatry 118: 403–406

Kolvin I, Humphrey M, McNay A (1971b) Studies in the childhood psychoses. VI. Cognitive factors in childhood psychoses. Br J Psychiatry 118: 415–419

Kolvin I, Ounsted C, Humphrey M, McNay A (1971c) Studies in the childhood psychoses. II. The phenomenology of childhood psychoses. Br J Psychiatry 118: 385–395

Kolvin I, Ounsted C, Richardson LM, Garside RF (1971d) Studies in the childhood psychoses. III. The family and social background in childhood psychoses. Br J Psychiatry 118: 396–402

Kolvin I, Ounsted C, Roth M (1971e) Studies in the childhood psychoses. V. Cerebral dysfunction and childhood psychoses. Br J Psychiatry 118: 407–414

Kraepelin E (1893) Ein kurzes Lehrbuch für Studierende und Ärzte, 4. Aufl. Abel, Leipzig

Kremen WS, Buka SL, Seidman LJ, Goldstein JM, Koren D, Tsuang MT (1998) IQ decline during childhood and adult psychotic symptoms in a community sample: a 19-year longitudinal study. Am J Psychiatry 155: 672–677

Leonhard K (1986) Aufteilung der endogenen Psychosen und ihre differenzierte Ätiologie, 6. Aufl. Akademie-Verlag, Berlin

Mahler MS (1952) On child psychosis and schizophrenia: autistic and symbiotic infantile psychosis. Psychoanal Study Child 7: 286–305

Mahler MS, Ross JR, de Fries Z (1949) Clinical studies in benign and malignant cases of childhood psychosis (schizophrenia-like). Am J Orthopsychiatry 19: 295–304

Martin M (1991) Der Verlauf der Schizophrenie im Jugendalter unter Rehabilitationsbedingungen. Enke, Stuttgart

McKenna K, Gordon C, Lenane M, Kaysen D, Fahey K, Rapoport J (1994) Looking for childhood onset schizophrenia: the first 71 cases screened. J Am Acad Child Adolesc Psychiatry 33: 636–644

Merry SN, Werry JS (2001) Course and prognosis. In: Remschmidt H (ed) Schizophrenia in children and adolescents. Cambridge University Press, Cambridge, pp 268–297

Modestin J, Sonderegger P, Erni T (2001) Follow-up study of hysterical psychosis, reactive, psychogenic psychosis and schizophrenia. Compr Psychiatry 42: 51–56

Rapoport JL, Giedd J, Jacobsen LK et al. (1997) Childhood-onset schizophrenia: progressive ventricular enlargement during adolescence on MRI brain re-scan. Arch Gen Psychiatry 54: 897–903

Remschmidt H, Brechtel B, Mewe F (1973) Zum Krankheitsverlauf und zur Persönlichkeitsstruktur von Kindern und Jugendlichen mit endogen-phasischen Psychosen und reaktiven Depressionen. Acta Paedopsychiatr 40: 2–17

Remschmidt H (1975a) Neuere Ergebnisse zur Psychologie und Psychiatrie der Adoleszenz. Z Kinder Jugendpsychiatr 3: 67–101

Remschmidt H (1975b) Psychologie und Psychopathologie der Adoleszenz. Monatsschr Kinderheilkunde 123: 316–323

Remschmidt H, Martin M, Schulz E, Gutenbrunner C, Fleischhaker C (1991) The concept of positive and negative schizophrenia in child and adolescent psychiatry. In: Marneros A, Andreasen NC, Tsuang MT (eds) Negative versus positive schizophrenia. Springer, Berlin Heidelberg New York, pp 219–242

Remschmidt H, Schulz E, Martin M, Warnke A, Trott GE (1994) Childhood onset schizophrenia: history of the concept and recent studies. Schizophr Bull 20: 727–745

Remschmidt H (ed) (2001) Schizophrenia in children and adolescents. Cambridge University Press, Cambridge

Remschmidt H, Martin M, Hennighausen K, Schulz E (2001) Treatment and rehabilitation. In: Remschmidt H (ed) Schizophrenia in children and adolescents. Cambridge University Press, Cambridge, pp 192–267

Remschmidt H (2002) Early-onset schizophrenia as a progressive-deteriorating developmental disorder: evidence from child psychiatry. J Neural Transm 109: 101–117

Remschmidt H, Martin M, Fleischhaker C, Schulz E (2005) A 42-year follow-up study of childhood-onset schizophrenia (unpublished)

Rutter M (1967) Psychotic disorders in early childhood. In: Coppen AJ, Walk A (eds) Recent developments in schizophrenia. Hedly Brothers, Ashford, pp 133–158

Schourfield J, McGuffin P (2001) Genetic aspects. In: Remschmidt H (ed) Schizophrenia in children and adolescents. Cambridge University Press, Cambridge, pp 119–134

Stutte H (1969) Psychosen des Kindesalters. In: Schmied F, Asperger H (eds) Neurologie – Psychologie – Psychiatrie. Springer, Berlin, pp 908–938 (Handb Kinderheilkunde, vol VIII/1)

Towbin K, Dykens E, Pearson G, Cohen D (1993) Conceptualizing "borderline syndrome of childhood" and "childhood schizophrenia" as a developmental disorder. J Am Acad Child Adolesc Psychiatry 32: 775–782

van der Gaag R (1993) Multiplex developmental disorder. Thesis, University of Utrecht

Werry JS, McClellan JM, Chard L (1991) Childhood and adolescent schizophrenia, bipolar and schizoaffective disorder: a clinical and outcome study. J Am Acad Child Adolesc Psychiatry 30: 457–465

Werry JS (1992) Child and adolescent (early-onset) schizophrenia: a review in the light of DSM-III-R. J Autism Dev Disord 22: 601–624

Werry JS, McClellan JM, Andrews LK, Hamm M (1994) Clinical features and outcome of child and adolescent schizophrenia. Schizophr Bull 20: 619–630

Wolff S (1995) Loners. The life path of unusual children. Routledge, London New York

Authors' address: H. Remschmidt, Department of Child and Adolescent Psychiatry, Philipps-University, Hans-Sachs-Strasse 6, 35033 Marburg, Germany, e-mail: remschm@med.uni-marburg.de